Living the RAW LIVE VEGAN Lifestyle

Finally, eat more and lose weight with optimal nutrition!

Susan Eugenie Rubarth

www.RawLiveVegan.com

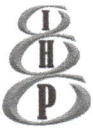

INTERNATIONAL HEALTH PUBLISHING
Carrollton, Texas, USA

INTERNATIONAL HEALTH PUBLISHING
February 22, 2008
Publishing Group Affirming Truth & Innate Wisdom

Copyright © 2012 by Susan Eugenie Rubarth
Image copyright © 2012 by Susan Eugenie Rubarth

First International Health Publishing trade paperback edition April 2012

All rights reserved, including the right of reproduction in whole or in part in any form or by any means, electronic or mechanical, including photocopy, recording, or any information storage and retrieval system, without written permission from the publisher, author, and copyright owners; except by a reviewer who may quote brief passages in review.

For information about special discounts for bulk purchase, please contact International Health Publishing at writer@InternationalHealthPublishing.com.

International Health Publishing can bring authors to your live events.
To book an event contact writer@InternationalHealthPublishing.com, or visit our website: www.InternationalHealthPublishing.com.

Living The Raw Live Vegan Lifestyle
Finally, eat more and lose weight with optimal nutrition!

Susan Eugenie Rubarth
www.RawLiveVegan.com

ISBN-13 978-0-9818353-7-2
ISBN-10 0-9818353-7-6

Library of Congress Control Number: 2011945591

SAN   856-6925

E-Pub ISBN-13 978-0-9818353-8-9
E-Pub ISBN-10 0-9818353-8-4

Manufactured in the United States of America, and printed on the finest 100% postconsumer-waste recycled paper

10 9 8 7 6 5 4 3 2 1

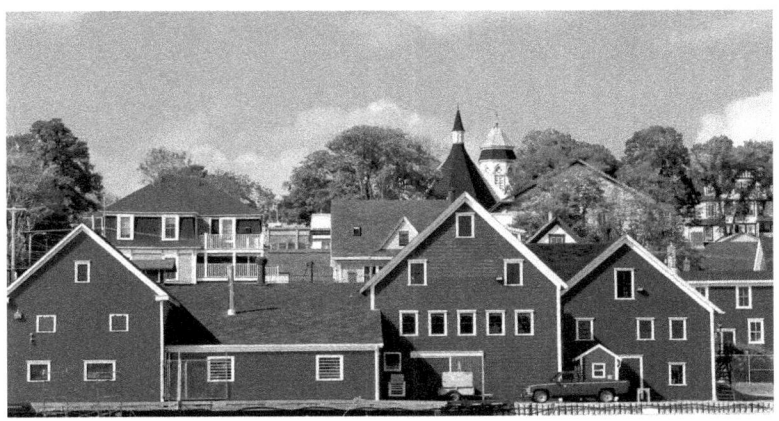

Dedication

This book is dedicated to my husband Phil, the love and joy that is my life. Thank you for believing in me, you inspire me to move beyond my comfort level, you are living proof of our chosen lifestyle. You are a willing partner in all things healthy.

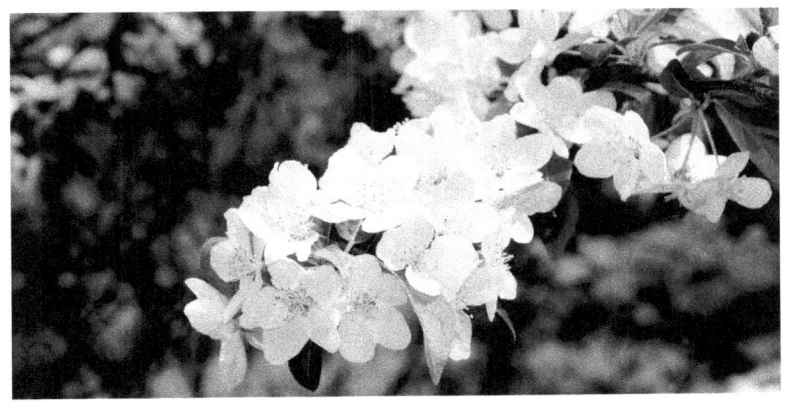

Acknowledgements

First of all I want to thank my son Bryan for his masterful photography in getting the right shot of the finished product for our recipes and for his time devoted to www.rawlivevegan.com.

Regarding nutrition, the Universe continues to feed me information through the people and books I come in contact with. My happenstance meeting of the following powerful women has not only touched but has been integral in my life, making me who I am today.

Andrea Hines imparted her knowledge on the topic of nutrition that transformed my life in such a profound way – thank you!

Glenna Jenkins saw the importance of my work and encouraged me to move beyond the raw live vegan site and write this book. Her edits and critiques combined with the designwork of Liz Hardy are the polish on the raw material – pardon the pun – thank you!

Dena Churchill, not allowing me to quit when I was discouraged, saw the importance of this book and so kindly recommended International Health Publishing, where Dr. Elizabeth Pilicy reviewed and agreed to publish *Living The Raw Live Vegan Lifestyle*. I am so very grateful!

Lastly, my Mother and my family, thank you for always believing there was more to me than met the eye.

The Universe does deliver when we are open to receiving it. While sometimes it is just a whisper, we must be silent to hear it – for this I am forever grateful!

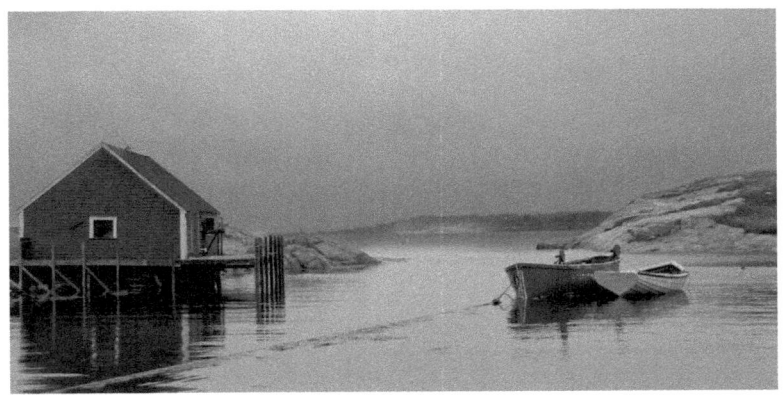

Foreword

Serendipity occurs when one accidentally stumbles upon something wonderful, when searching for something else. This serendipitous moment, for us, occurred during the pursuit of optimum health. After searching for solutions to my and my husband's health problems, I found Dr. William LaValley.

Author's Journey Into Wellness

Sometimes we feel as if no one is listening. And even though we try our best to be our own health advocates when seeking answers to what ails us, we feel very much alone, particularly when we have limited time with our physician.

My personal interest has always been health. I have a library full of books to prove it, many of which have stood the test of time. They cover such topics as nutrition, pH balance, hormones and aging. They formed the bases of my own research and continuing quest to age healthfully. They provided the link to optimal health that my husband, Phil, and I enjoy today. And they are part of the building blocks of the Raw Live Vegan program that I developed over the past three years and am now sharing with you.

In my thirties, I taught weight management classes as I wanted to help people understand the basics of good nutrition, lose weight and regain their health. I soon found that the program I taught was only effective for the general population below age forty. For women, especially, losing those last few pounds and achieving their goal weight was almost impossible. Despite keeping meticulous journals and reporting in every week, some lost little or no weight, others gained. Frustrated, they turned to their general practitioners for guidance in selecting a realistic goal weight that would receive the blessing of the weight management organization I worked for. The new goals, for age and height, set by their doctors were much higher than the targets set by my organization. I was later to find that other critical measures of health had also been raised. These included hormone levels, blood pressure and blood sugars, to name a few. These new targets accommodated the majority of our present North American population that could not achieve the previous lower ones due to a diet based on foods available in today's marketplace.

In my endeavors to help these women, I studied journals provided to me by my employer. I wanted to gain some insight as to why they were having difficulties losing weight and why some continued to gain weight despite strict adherence to the program in both diet and exercise. These women had become frustrated with their low caloric, high-energy output, which are actually a paradox when you think about it and a fast track to illness. In hindsight, I realize that my lack of knowledge was the missing piece to the puzzle. It wasn't until I reached my forties and was no longer teaching the program when I found myself facing the same dilemma. Despite a healthy diet and regular exercise, the weight crept on. By age 50 I hit the top of the weight chart for my age and height. So there I was, far removed from my role as a weight loss coach, finding that I WAS THAT 50 YEAR OLD WOMAN sitting in my weight management class, with a carefully written journal, filled out right down to the last glass of water. Now I was gaining the weight. I was that woman begging for insight into weight control. It was then that I began my quest for optimal health.

In my nursing program, which I embarked on when my children were grown, I studied a variety of topics. Among them were the two states of acidosis and alkalosis, which cause our electrolytes to go out of balance and compromise kidney and heart function. I wondered what caused these imbalances and found that it was poor nutrition. I researched further and started putting the pieces together on my own by using what I had learned in my nursing program as a foundation and reading beyond the recommended curriculum to fill in the gaps.

I learned that our internal systems work like a finely tuned engine when properly nourished. But when we burden them with chemically- laden, processed convenience foods that are high in calories, fat, sodium and preservatives they begin to malfunction. The delicate balance of pH, which is maintained through proper nutrition, becomes compromised. Good health requires that our systems are alkaline.

My own state of health and my work as a health care professional led me to realize that our health care system is overburdened from treating the ill effects of bad nutrition. At 50 I found myself unacceptably overweight. I was also entering peri-menopause (now there's a time bomb), and didn't know when I would be going from peri- to flat out menopause. One day I found myself standing in front of a mirror, in the privacy of my bathroom, nude. I didn't like what I saw. Gone was the lithe, girlish figure of my former youth. Over it laid the results of ten years of aging. My body had changed in a negative way, despite my hard efforts at diet and exercise. I was miserable. At the same time, menopause was fast approaching, with it, a variety of symptoms, some physical, some emotional. I lacked energy; had low libido; and had gained weight. I also had dry itchy skin; psoriasis on my elbows; cracked skin on my heels, despite regular pedicures; and cracked fingernails. I had brain fog during the day, and caught myself falling asleep. Oddly enough, I had trouble sleeping at night. I had muscle and joint pain. I lacked motivation to exercise. And when I did exercise, I no longer had that euphoric feeling I once knew after a good workout. And often times, I was such an emotional wreck that I would cry or fly off the handle over nothing.

My husband, Phil, on the other hand, had always appeared to be healthy. He had put on some weight over the years and, lucky for him, that it was evenly distributed. But it was his family's history of high cholesterol and diabetes that caused me concern. Phil's cholesterol had elevated. I also suspected that his healthy outward appearance masked a number of other ailments due to his twenty- eight years working in the construction industry. At middle age, Phil and I both found our selves in less than optimal health despite our best efforts in good nutrition and plenty of exercise.

As a family, we ate healthfully. Our diet was mainly Mediterranean. We ate plenty of fruits and vegetables, whole natural grains, fish and lean meats. Lunches and dinners included a salad. Dressings were made with olive oil, which was also used for cooking. Any baked goods I made myself, again from whole grains. When grocery shopping I stayed away from soda pop, chips and pre-packaged foods. We did not consume processed foods of any kind. But we did partake of low fat microwave popcorn, and yes, this is junk too! Through all of this my weight yo-yoed from the top of the range for my age and height, to the middle and back up again, despite my careful diet. I questioned my thyroid, I questioned my hormones, I questioned everything medical as I knew that what went past my lips was healthy, or so the food industry would have me believe. My husband, on the other hand, maintained that if our doctor said we were healthy, who were we to differ?

Despite my concerns, my physician assured me that as I was within the healthy range for weight, cholesterol and blood pressure I shouldn't worry. According to him, my symptoms were all part of the natural aging process. Most women at this stage of life are in an emotional state due to hormonal imbalance and accept a medication that manages the emotional state but unfortunately has the side effect of lowered metabolic rate that in the end compounds her health problem.

I raged quietly on the inside, while trying to hold it together. I had gone to my medical appointment armed with my food/activity journal, current cutting edge information on nutrition and hormonal imbalance and old pictures of myself, trying to figure out how I could go from 125 pounds in my early thirties to 170 pounds at fifty and still be considered healthy. Now this man was suggesting that I had a problem accepting a natural aging process. To my doctor, I was just another hormonally unbalanced woman, the outer office was full of patients near death's door and my fifteen minutes were up.

When I thought about his opinion on my health issues – that there really were none, I started to second guess myself. I wondered if I was just another one of those baby boomers given to vanity. I wondered if I had become a part of the 'all about me' generation looking for a magic pill. But, when I really thought about it, I came to the conclusion that it is difficult to get to the problem, when your doctor doesn't perceive there to be one in the first place. I knew then that my expectations for my own health and for my husband's did not fit within his traditional 'wait and see' approach. Fifteen minutes is simply not long enough to discuss blood work, to review the information that I had brought to the table and to discuss my past history. When I left his office, with my journal and a raft of information that I had with me, that he did not have time to discuss, I knew I was on my own.

My doctor was a kind man, and I understand him to be very good in his field. I am grateful to him for good care in the past. But as he is schooled in a certain pharmaceutically based belief system and not well versed in alternative medicine, we did not understanding each other on my health issues. It became abundantly clear to me that I was looking for something that he could not provide. I also knew, by then, that the answers to my health dilemma could be found in nutrition and hormones.

I had already started collecting the information I felt necessary to achieve personal wellness. I understood that I had to become totally self-reliant for everything that had to do with my health with the exception of hormone replacement therapy. And in my quest for greater personal wellness, I simply closed the door on conventional medicine.

We will always have conventional, pharmaceutically based medicine, just as we will always have alternative medicine. They each serve a purpose. They also, generally, serve two different camps. I am a firm believer in both types of medicine. But I want to address my own personal wellness program as naturally as I can, through nutrition and natural therapies first. If I do this then, in the event that I need pharmaceuticals, I will be in the best possible shape to benefit from them. And as long as we have people feeding themselves unhealthily, we will need conventional medicine to control their related conditions. Many people manage their health through pharmaceuticals. They eat and drink whatever they want to and tweak their medications as required. Others take their nutrition seriously and avoid many of the common ailments that result from a poor diet by respecting and understanding what they are putting into their bodies.

As alternative medicine is where I found success for my own health and also for the health of my family, I continued to study more on the subject of nutrition, in general, and how it effects aging. I learned more through my own personal study than I did in my nursing program. Nutrition was a small component of my program that centered on the Canada Food Guide. And despite the fact that the food pyramid in the Guide has changed drastically over the years, we still face an increasingly obese population.

In my quest to learn, I found that low energy and weight gain are mainly caused by hormone depletion, even when on a healthy diet. Combine hormonal imbalance with the current unhealthy North American diet of inferior processed foods and this spells disaster. For most women, menopause and hormone depletion will continue to be ignored, whereas it should be a major health concern. Our mothers and grandmothers all journeyed through menopause. They were forced to do so 'naturally' as there were no treatments. This does not necessarily mean that they coped well. Many didn't. Hormone imbalance can cause depression and mood swings. And what about the husbands and children who lived with these women? How did they cope? Hormone replacement relieves afflicted women of these conditions. Bio-identical hormones are specifically tailored to individual hormonal conditions and they restore balance.

My New Year's Resolution for 2009 was for Phil and I to achieve the optimal health that would permit us to age gracefully and enjoy the next fifty years. Between January and May of 2009, I read fourteen books on nutrition, aging, hormones and wellness. In the pages of the many books I read I learned about compounding pharmaceuticals, bio-identical hormones, organic health supplements, current food guides and the sorry state of health in our current population. I learned about the direct benefits that certain foods have on our health, and how they can relieve symptoms of menopause. I learned that if our hormones were out of balance, then everything else was too. These studies in nutrition and hormonal imbalance validated my feelings and made me feel sane again. For some women their approach to transitioning through menopause will be *au-naturel*. I laude those who can transition naturally through this difficult stage in aging, but I knew that it wasn't for me. For me the importance of nutrition in enhancing hormonal balance with the possible supplementation of bio-identical hormones if necessary would be key in making this anything but natural transition easy and comfortable. Many books pointed to bio-identical hormones attributing to many women's resilience, restoration and rejuvenation.

All of the physicians, whose books I had read, agreed on the benefits of bio-identical hormones. These physicians also agreed that past studies on hormone replacement therapies and breast cancer were flawed. These studies were based on women taking hormonal therapy, the chemically produced *Premarin*, which is derived from the urine of pregnant mares. Bio-identical hormones are not produced this way. Finally, all of these books and seminars on the aging process noted that this stage in life could be wonderful, but only if we retrain ourselves on nutrition and discard our many bad habits. After all of this investigation, I felt that I was sitting at a table with a large monochromatic puzzle, that the pieces were there, and it was up to me to find out how they went together. But at least I had found the pieces.

In the spring of 2009, I attended a seminar on hormonal imbalance and bio-identical hormones in Dartmouth, Nova Scotia, sponsored by a local compounding pharmacy, *Moffatt's*. Dr. Kenna Stevenson, an American physician and the author of *Awakening Athena*, was the keynote speaker. Dr. Stevenson had presented a number of sold out seminars throughout the province. She even offered a dinner/seminar to local family physicians, but it was poorly attended. The few that were present did not seem interested in the topic, I suspect because bio-identical hormone replacement therapies are not produced by "Big Pharma," as it is a natural product that cannot be patented.

Doctors today are more apt to prescribe *Premarin* or other nonhuman and artificial human hormones. The problem with *Premarin* is that it is produced from the urine of pregnant mares; the estrogen doesn't match human estrogen.

The Women's Health Initiative, published in the Journal of the National Cancer Institute, states that the risks of being on *Premarin* are increasing. The latest findings are that it can cause benign proliferative breast disease, which can potentially cause malignancies. Other known risks are ovarian cancer, heart attack, stroke, blood clots and gall bladder disease. But the pharmaceutical industry has nothing to offer as an acceptable therapy for women experiencing difficulties during menopause. The only alternative offered by the pharmaceutical industry is no treatment at all.

Some women do go through menopause naturally, with little discomfort and few side effects. They might gain a little weight, feel a bit tired and experience a hot flash or two. But this is the minority. So do we base our beliefs on what we can tolerate on the experience of a minority of women? I think not. Many, like myself, have felt like a finely knit sweater raveling in all directions. Hormonal imbalance can strike at any time. We need to educate our daughters and ourselves on its signs and symptoms. Hormonal imbalance can cause weight gain, reduced energy, emotional swings, depression, psychosis, brain fog, poor concentration, loss of libido, night sweats and difficulty sleeping, among others. The list is long.

Many women in my age group with the same symptoms and complaints are on anti- depressants. The sad fact is these pills only make you feel better over the short term. These are 'managed feelings.' And as anti- depressants slow everything down, including the metabolic rate, the side effect is weight gain - lovely!

Another area of conventional medicine I find problematic is how it determines healthy weight. Charts that present a cookie- cutter approach to health for the masses are deceiving. Measures they tell us to strive for are not necessarily healthy for everyone as they attempt to pigeonhole entire groups according to age, height and gender. Tables that discuss weight ranges according to sex and height can be totally misconstrued by your doctor and or yourself. People are not all alike. Weight ranges can vary by as much as forty pounds depending on body type. You can start at the low end of the range when you are young, gain weight as you age, and still be at the low end at middle age even when you know that you, personally, are overweight. The same can be said for the BMI chart. These charts have huge variances and they do not consider a person's bone structure, activity level and metabolic rate. In my case, my doctor saw me as female, 50 years of age, peri-menopausal, and still within the range set by Health Canada, with no consideration for my past history and how I had gone from the bottom to the top of the chart, through the aging process. Believe me, this is one range you don't want to be at the top of!

From my personal experience I knew that conventional medicine did not have the answers that I sought. From my reading, I suspected that part of my problem was hormonal, and if this was the case, then I had to make hormonal changes and I had to make them soon. I was already approaching peri-menopause and the clock was ticking. From a nutritional level, I was at a loss, as I discovered that everything that I knew to be true about food had been a lie. The food industry, with its chemically laden additives, and products with infinite shelf life, never mind the toxic packaging, was killing us.

By this time I was determined that Phil and I would age gracefully. I also wanted us to avoid the genetic pitfalls that befell other family members without the use of prescription drugs. But the way we were feeling, at the time, said that we were heading in this precarious direction. And if we wanted to continue being active participants of life and not spectators, we knew that we had to make a dramatic nutritional shift and we had to make it fast. With these lofty objectives, I knew we needed a new doctor. So, I sought a foreword-thinking professional, who was versed in the same alternative health practices that I had been studying. He or she would have to be someone who would listen to our concerns and help guide us as we worked toward our goals. In May 2009, five months after our New Year's resolutions, Luckily, I found a doctor just twenty minutes away. I immediately booked an appointment with Dr. William LaValley.

Before our first appointment with Dr. LaValley, he sent us for blood work and asked us to fill out a questionnaire entailing in-depth medical history and return it him. He wanted to understand some of our health issues before meeting us. We were impressed by the level of organization taken before our initial appointment; and even more impressed when he listened to our concerns and reviewed our histories. Finally, we had found the doctor who understood us.

Dr. LaValley supported my husband and I in our pursuit of optimal health. He shared his knowledge of healthy aging through nutrition, natural hormones and supplements tailored to our specific needs. He agreed that a healthy diet, hormonal balance and exercise are inseparable components to optimal health. He helped us move through a maze of new information and was open to concepts we brought to the table, provided they were backed by sound research. He monitored our health through regular blood work and charted our successes. He reviewed my journal, which included details of the wide variety of foods I consumed, the moods I experienced and the amount of activity I enjoyed. I also kept detailed notes of my monthly menstrual cycles. He noted the increased activity I now enjoyed. These health-related successes inspired me to develop the Raw Live Vegan program. It was this program that transported Phil and I from constant fatigue to optimal health.

Developing this program to address our nutritional needs required organization. I needed to accumulate a variety of ingredients and buy different appliances. Retraining the brain to not cook food or heat it up on days that dip below freezing was a test of strength. Knowing that I had to understand how to include a variety of organic fruits and vegetables, raw grains, nuts and beans, I had to learn a whole new way to prepare food, how to sprout, store and grow. I had to source anything that could not be bought in our small community of 2500 people or one of the other small towns nearby. At first, it was a tad overwhelming. Then it became inspiring. This is when I developed my website and started to write this book, I wanted to simplify the transition for others wanting to adopt this lifestyle to achieve optimal health. Residing in Canada's unhealthiest town, according to Best Health, a Canadian Magazine, motivated me to achieve optimal health and to show others that they can too!

I would be lying if I said that I wasn't overwhelmed. The whole process of my journey was a great deal of work. But when I think back to the day I stood naked peering with self-loathing and misery in that mirror at a body I no longer recognized, I know it was all worth it. Phil and I have turned back the hands of time. Thanks to the Raw Live Vegan lifestyle we now have strong, healthy bodies. Optimal health cannot be had from starvation and exercise; there is so much more involved. The key to any success is knowledge. This lifestyle will only work if you adhere to all of its components. You must be patient in learning all of the components involved in raw live vegan. It will seem difficult at first; but believe me it will be worth it!

The research I have done has given me a solid base of knowledge in alternative health. My findings are backed by legitimate research. I have earned the respect of many in the field. My program is solid. It works.

Keep in mind that if you are overweight and unhealthy, the fault is not your own. It can be shared by the food industry that fills the center aisles of our grocery store. These are the foods that are easy to prepare. They have an infinite shelf life. And the majority of them contain most of the ingredients that are the root cause of our health-related problems.

Contents

ONE	Raw Live Vegan for the Health Of It!	1
TWO	Let's Get Started	12
THREE	Appliances & Their Benefits	83
FOUR	Not Just Your Average Food!	92
FIVE	Taking Food Knowledge to The Next Level	125
SIX	Three Keys To Success	148
SEVEN	Habits Worth Forming	168
EIGHT	Motivation	185
NINE	Eyes Wide Open	202
TEN	MENU Planners	209
ELEVEN	Recipes	242
	Breakfast Ideas	242
	Lunches & Light Fare	248
	Main Meals	256
	Breads & Crackers	273
	Dips & Spreads	278
	Dressings, Sauces & Condiments	281
	Desert	285
	Appetizers & Snacks	294
	Beverages	300
TWELVE	In Closing	303
	Bibliography	310
	Author's Background	313

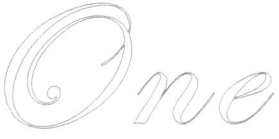

Raw Live Vegan
For The Health Of It!

Raw Live Vegan Lifestyle Defined

Raw live vegan is the purest form of vegan. Raw denotes not cooked, Live denotes enzymes and nutrients still viable, as close to organically fresh picked plant-based produce – from garden to table! Vegan, of course, means nothing from animal but everything plant-based. This diet excludes all food of animal origin and does not cook any of its food above 118 degrees Fahrenheit/48 degrees Celsius. Foods enjoyed are plant-based foods of fruit, vegetables, grains, nuts, seeds and legumes. Limiting, you ask? Hardly – the variety of foods associated with this lifestyle are endless.

Raw live vegan is easy to define; can the same be said about us? Are we any of the labels society thoughtlessly pins on us? Such as apple or pear-shaped? Now there's a picture. Please don't be offended; I was considered by the medical profession to be pear-shaped. There's more, I should be grateful – as pear-shaped figures are healthier than apple-shaped figures! According to those in the know, apple-shaped figures may be at greater risk of cardiovascular disease and diabetes, to name a couple! Pear-shaped individuals may be at risk of osteoporosis, varicose veins and blood clots. Grateful to be a *pear*? I think not! I was not born a *pear*, thank you very much! When my physicality on the inside and the outside was changing for the worse, I was less than accepting and refused to be defined as a "mature female-subject failing to accept the aging process..." Despite doubling my caloric intake, I regained my inner and outer vitality and youthful physique in rapid time – and without the feeling of lethargy, cravings, etc. As for the varicose veins, I did have the beginning signs in one leg and nipped that in the bud (more on this in the last chapter of this book). As for the osteoporosis, I have a bone density examination every five years and am happy to say that my bones are at an optimal state with no signs of osteoporosis. This is thanks to the raw live vegan lifestyle, coupled with my desire to exercise with the excessive energy I have from eating well. Knowing the choice is yours to make, how will you define yourself?

What pulled me into this lifestyle was definitely health-issue related; however, the tasty recipes are what kept me. It was an added bonus to know I was doing my body a world-of-good! Most assume it is salad alone, followed by an actual fruit for dessert; this is an option but how about Greek Pizza, with a side order of yummy appetizers and perhaps "Ice Kream" for dessert! Pure basic organic foods can be made into miraculous meals without the guilt!

The reasons to consider this lifestyle are plentiful. If you suffer from obesity, high blood pressure, hypertension or inflammation you should give this lifestyle a second look! Many studies attribute favorable results by adopting the various components of this lifestyle. My personal aim in this book is not only to share the rapid successes toward optimal health my husband and I have achieved, moreover it is to dismiss the fear of change and the attitude that it is difficult to have a healthy lifestyle. I will prove this lifestyle is as easy as child's play!

> "I want to help you understand your addictions surrounding food, understand your slowed metabolic rate, understand your current lack of energy. It can be corrected with "FOOD," not the lack of, the secret is in the choices and what really is in the food being marketed to you as *healthy*."

Benefits of Raw Live Vegan Lifestyle!

Real food, high energy, optimal health and longevity – these are just some of the benefits! Our grandparents enjoyed the secret to a long life. They found it in the nutritious, wholesome, unprocessed foods they ate. Oftentimes, they grew it themselves. Before the days of refrigeration they too dehydrated a lot of their crops to enjoy later in the winter months. Somehow, we have moved away from this healthy lifestyle, into one that is fast-paced and competitive. In the process, we embraced a diet that is highly processed, chemically laden with infinite shelf life all in the name of convenience. We often eat on the fly, rarely taking the time to prepare a nutritious, well-balanced meal to share with our families around the dinner table. Instead, we choose processed foods that we pop into the oven or the microwave or worse, pick up at the drive-through of a fast food outlet. Despite all of this, we consider ourselves to be *healthy*, at least by today's standards. Yet the typical North American diet leads to high cholesterol, diabetes, heart disease, and cancer. Food is a powerful tool. It has the ability to make us sick or to cure us. Even in today's busy world, we shall be conscious of the importance of nutritious food and of the way we prepare it. A healthy menu includes fruits, vegetables, fibre, protein and hydration on a daily basis. Include "superfoods" for a nutritional boost in health. They are nutrient dense, antioxidant rich, disease fighting, anti-aging and, yes, beautifying. They also enhance wellbeing and boost the immune system. Check out the section on Superfoods in chapter four.

The foods we use in the Raw Live Vegan program help trim and revitalize the body. They are not preserved, processed, pasteurized, adulterated or irradiated. They are not baked, boiled, braised, barbequed or microwaved. Most of our recipes focus on the RAW aspect of food preparation. Raw foods contain enzymes that aid in digestion and are readily absorbed into the bloodstream. To achieve optimal uptake we must take our time chewing our food to actually break down the cell structure of the raw plant-based food. This is why juicing is superior for breaking down cell structure making the nutrients readily available for absorption without the chewing. Check out our section on Juicing. Looking back into the history of food, we find that traditional meals in many cultures opened with a salad, as the fresh, raw, live aspect of this dish aided in the digestion of courses that followed.

The majority of raw foods are alkaline (basic), which is very important for optimal pH balance. Acidic, chemically laden, high fat, high sugar cooked or processed foods have been linked to many diseases that most consider natural in the aging process.

Raw food may not cure all aliments, but it will do far more for your body than a high fat, high sugar, processed diet. Food is never cooked at temperatures above 118 degrees Fahrenheit. Temperatures above this kill the natural enzymes that boost your body's immune system and help it fight off disease. Mindful eaters who enjoy Raw Live Vegan food are not all 100% RAW Foodies. But all will affirm that the more RAW the better, simply because when you overcook food, you destroy the vitamins and nutrients. If it is heat you want, get it through spices, or warm it up to 118 degrees Fahrenheit/48 degrees Celsius.

Going 80% RAW Live Vegan is a realistic goal. This book introduces you to the various aspects of the Raw Live Vegan lifestyle. If you have just started the program, you are on the right path. Check into our website often (www.rawlivevegan.com) to read our new articles, try our new recipes, and continue to reap the rewards gained by eating raw food.

Raw Live Vegan Is Affordable

A household budget is a list of discretionary and nondiscretionary expenditures we make every month balanced against monthly income. Nondiscretionary expenses are items we have little control over, such as the mortgage or rent, water, electricity, and insurance. We can call this the 'non-choices' part of our budget as we need these items and can usually count on them costing the same every month. Discretionary expenses are items we have more control over. We can also call this the 'choices' part of our budget as it lists the items that we need or want, and the amount of money we spend on them reflects our personal choices and lifestyle. These items include cable TV, telephone/internet, recreation, clothing, charities, entertainment, savings and food. The 'choices' part of our budget is used as a guideline for what we can and cannot afford. It also lists expenses according to priority, so that during tight months unnecessary expenses can be cut. The common belief is that healthy eating cannot be supported on a tight budget. But when you consider the 'choices' part of your budget, this does not have to be so, as frivolous *wants* can be replaced by healthful *needs*.

When thinking about budgets, the Raw Live Vegan program has definite advantages. Most of the food on the program can be purchased in bulk and stored over long periods of time. Beans, grains, nuts, seeds and spices can be purchased in bulk. And for some items, the more you buy the less you pay per pound. All of these items have a long shelf life, which can be extended in the freezer. If your freezer is energy smart, you can take advantage of sales and stock up. Coconut milk, for example, is an excellent buy when on sale, and it freezes well. Also, check out canned organic products that periodically go on sale and stock up your pantry.

Buying local and in season saves money too. Fall is an excellent time to buy bulk organic fruits and vegetables directly from the farmer. You can freeze or dehydrate them for further use. Bartering is a great way to save money. If you are a gardener consider growing the crops that thrive in your garden and swapping with another gardener. This way two or more of you can benefit from a wider variety of fresh fruits and vegetables. Some gardeners even swap flowers or honey for fruits and vegetables. If you know someone with a large piece of unused land, consider approaching him or her with the idea of starting a community garden. You are only as limited as your resourcefulness.

Making your own products is a great money saver and it's healthier, too. You can make your own almond milk with soaked almonds, water and a good blender. You can make your own almond flour with a good blender that has a dry blade or a good food processor. I tend to grind my own flax flour knowing that it is fresher. Rather than buy my bean sprouts, I sprout them. I make my own humus, in bulk, in a food processor. I also make my own raw-organic-crackers and breakfast bread in my dehydrator. For me time is money, so I make a huge batch of humus, and 10-racks of crackers and bread at a time and freeze them. I soak my oat groats, barley and buckwheat for my morning cereal instead of buying pre-packaged cereals from health food sections. The more I do myself, the more I save. Think back to olden days when our pioneering grandparents emigrated from other countries and did not have access to a corner store. Our forefathers had pantries filled with good, nutritious food that could be turned into epicurean delights to feed the family and the farmhands. This was affordable too!

If you are still thinking that all of this costs money, then evaluate your present lifestyle; check your budget and you will soon see items that can be replaced by healthy food. Perhaps this could be something as simple as reviewing your latest grocery receipt and adding up all of the money spent on pre-packaged, process foods. You may have to look no further than the ice cream you just bought that was far more expensive than the bananas that just went on sale. Frozen bananas and maple syrup with a few nuts on top are not only cheaper than ice cream, they are healthier and they taste better too. I scour the produce section and when I see a good buy on organic bananas, I buy in bulk and freeze them.

If you buy your lunch at work, consider bringing healthier lunches from home. You will soon find that you are not only saving money, but you are saving time too. While your co-workers are waiting for their own food in a cramped cafeteria, you will have already enjoyed yours and found time for a walk outdoors before returning to work. And what about the network charges for your TV? Perhaps you could consider reducing the number of channels you pay for. This would have the added benefit of getting you off of the couch, giving you more time for exercise.

Is there money invested in extra vehicles with extra insurance costs that you could sell, so that you can use the funds for healthier needs? The appliances that we need in order to transition into this lifestyle can be affordable too. If you want a particular appliance you could consider asking for it as a gift for a special occasion. Or you can sell off appliances that you will no longer be using, such as that deep fat fryer, sandwich maker, ice-cream maker, popcorn maker, etc. Why not look for appliances in the used, reconditioned or second hand section of newspapers, or source them on-line.

Keeping in mind that your health is your wealth, you will see that by adopting a healthier lifestyle your dependency on pharmaceuticals will become a thing of the past. This will save you money too. Any change can be scary to the novice. But as you make your transition, you will be able to dispel all the myths that say going Raw Live Vegan is expensive. Poor health costs much, much more.

Some great free on-line resources include: www.rawlivevegan.com, www.naturalnews.com, www.thehormonediet.com, to name just a few. Be careful about the source you choose as you will find that there is good and bad information everywhere. Our www.rawlivevegan.com is a free subscription site and information source that explains the multifaceted approach to optimal health. It puts the onus on you, the reader, to change your dietary habits through planning, selective shopping and careful food preparation.

Transitioning Into Raw Live Vegan

People assume to go raw live vegan is to give up certain foods forever and that a raw live vegan can never eat certain food groups like meat or dairy ever, ever again! Not the case! Most raw live vegans enjoy the lifestyle and practice an 80% adherence to the recommended foods, thereby leaving 20%

of their food intake to choose from foods, even foods from the "Foods to Avoid" list. Some raw live vegans use their 20% to steam or cook a favorite vegan dish and never choose an animal based food, ultimately the choice is yours! Transition should be fun and enjoyable! Not stressful!

The whole spirit of the Raw Live Vegan lifestyle is one of calm and serenity. You, like others before you, will happen upon your place of serenity within this program. Take baby steps and appreciate your efforts as you progress. Any good program should not be stressful. Stress is unhealthy for the GI tract, as when you are stressed your body will not absorb nutrients from the food you eat. So calm is key. I believe transitioning slowly is a benefit to the body so that you get used to the food slowly, as change to any type of diet creates change in the GI tract, some will witness diarrhea and cramping as their body becomes accustomed to handling a higher intake of raw vegetables and beans. Symptoms relating to gas will soon be a thing of the past, no pun intended.

You will meet those who wonder how far they can delve into the Raw Live Vegan lifestyle. The prospect of going 100% seems daunting. But consider this: if you ate a salad for lunch, using organic vegetables and the proper oil and vinegars with some onion bread (our recipe), you would be 30% RAW. Add a change to your breakfast routine by preparing one of our powerful shakes and a small bowl of soaked groats topped with maple syrup, a few soaked nuts and half of a banana together with lunch – you are now 60% RAW. How difficult is that! If you try some of our main meals for supper, something easy (they're all easy), such as the Marinara with Zucchini Noodles, you are up to 90% RAW for the day. You still have 10% left for your evening snack - early evening, that is, as late snacks disrupt sleep.

Relax with this plan and transition one day at a time. If you incorporate four raw main meals (lunches), leaving three main meals (suppers) to enjoy what your heart desires, you would then be at 85% RAW. And don't blame me if you start to lose your craving for meat.

While transitioning, you will begin to notice what others around you are doing. Some are adopting Raw Live Vegan as a lifestyle; some are following it 100% for a two weeks only cleanse; some venture into it more slowly, taking baby steps. Regardless of how they adapt to the program, they all share how great they feel and how well they sleep when they stay true to the program. You will become aware of organic issues. You will pick up on environmental issues. When dining out you will start to notice menu choices that fit nicely into your program. You are becoming totally aware and doing well for yourself.

You will become accustomed to the various places to shop within your community, even within your own local grocery store. You will notice that they too are aware of the movement toward healthy, organic eating and they do not want to lose that corner of the market. Some products, such as Yacan syrup, that may not be available at your local grocer or health food store, can be sourced on the Internet. The globe is at your fingertips, and you will quickly find a plethora of goods ready to ship.

So if you are interested in slowing down the signs of aging, regaining vitality, and restoring your health, there is no better way than Raw Live Vegan for instant, rapid results. As I transitioned from a healthy "Mediter-Asian" diet to this one, I was amazed at the fast results, not just for me but for my husband too. We both lost weight and regained vitality in no time at all. If this is your choice, concentrate on you. If others in your household are interested, then share the food and the labor. This transition into a healthy lifestyle is well worth the effort. This lifestyle is nutritionally sound for all ages and should be a point of pride in what you feed yourself and your loved ones. Remember, our health is our wealth. Without it, we have nothing!

> "Thank you for your kind and generous words regarding my participation in your wellness journey. The truth is: you both have chosen and continue to choose the activities to obtain and maintain increasingly better health. That's the big power of your actions - real healthy results and outcomes! You are living the daily choices and activities that demonstrate the practical reality of 'healthy input gives healthy results'. By providing people with a glimpse of how you are implementing these powerful choices in your lives, you give healing to many who would otherwise not get it. Your courage, tenacity, diligence, creativity and practical implementation will continue to give you both robust, durable healthy well-being. That is inspirational to me and to anyone interested in healthy well-being."
>
> ~ Dr. J. William LaValley

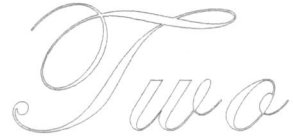

Let's Get Started

Allowable Food Lists & the Science Behind Them!

The hard facts behind the allowable food lists gives you great comfort knowing that the foods are not just a random, trendy choice, but are science based.

Water & Teas

As our body is made-up of 70% water, drinking plenty of it is vital to maintaining good health. When we exert ourselves and perspire, we need to rehydrate to maintain balance. As water has a perfect 7.0 pH, it is a natural gift that helps maintain proper pH balance. It bathes each of our cells and removes waste products from our GI tract. Start the day with one cup of water shortly after rising. Remember, we have gone all night without water. This rehydrates us and encourages stomach acid production to digest breakfast. The recommended daily amount is 6 to 8 cups, depending on our level of activity. The more active we are the more we perspire, so remember to keep hydrated. If we do not have the natural tendency to reach for a glass of water it may be due to possible dehydration. This causes our brain to stop sending signals that tell us to drink. In this case we may have to force ourselves to drink those 8 glasses a day. After a month

Let's Get Started

we will again have that signal firing from the brain telling us that we are thirsty.

Teas come in four basic varieties: black tea, green tea, white tea and oolong tea. These teas have fabulous medicinal properties; they boost the immune system, lower blood sugar and cholesterol, prevent tooth decay, slow the aging process, decrease high blood pressure, and prevent arthritis, stroke, heart disease, cancer and more. Added to this is the unlimited variety of herbal teas in the marketplace today. Flavors such as rum, toffee or tiramisu will satisfy you guilt free. Among my favorites are licorice, chocolate, ginger and orange. Some herbal teas have nutritional or medicinal benefits. When I feel under the weather, nothing is more soothing than a warm cup of chamomile tea. Check out the varieties at the local grocer, health food store or teashop.

On a recent trip to California, I stopped into a fabulous teashop called Dr. Tea's. It was a virtual tea emporium. As I wandered about, I met a tea server, offering a new blend of iced coffee tea. It tasted like crème caramel and it was absolutely incredible! The proprietor had developed a diet, based on teas, to aid people with specific health issues. The information I gained from this shop was not lost on me as my sister-in-law, Pauline, had already introduced our family to the benefits of beautiful herbal teas. Pauline's father grows tea in China. Every year we are the lucky recipients of his best loose green tea.

As tea leaves are dried at low temperatures, they are found on the alkaline side of the chart, unlike coffee beans, which are roasted at high temperatures. Several clinical studies have shown that green tea extract increases thermogenesis (the production of body heat) and fat oxidation (fats metabolized and used by the body to produce energy so it's not stored). It has been determined that the EGCG (epigallocatechin gallate) component in green tea has the greatest impact on fat loss. So when purchasing green tea make sure that it is standardized for EGCG. Green tea also has natural occurring caffeine, which is known to boost metabolic rate and energy. As the recommended daily amount is 3 cups (200mg) a day, space it out and enjoy its natural benefits. Those of us who like coffee can still enjoy one cup of organic coffee each day. It is good for us, as it promotes regularity and stimulates the liver to release toxins, so we should be able to easily fit it into our desired ratio of alkali/acid balance.

Hard core coffee drinkers, who know they need to cut back, but don't want the headaches associated with going cold turkey, can try black tea and transition slowly. Black tea contains half the caffeine of coffee. Its L-theanine neutralizes the harmful side effects of caffeine and is also known to act as an appetite suppressant. Green tea has half the caffeine of black tea, white tea has half the caffeine of green tea, and herbal tea has none. With our new, reduced caffeine intake we soon find our sleep pattern returning to that of a child.

Fruits

Fruit should make up 15% of our daily food intake.

Fruit should make up 15% of our daily intake. Check out the list and then enjoy the market for what is in season. Although buying local should be a priority, I do believe in fair trade and the benefits of a global economy. So I will buy that pineapple, which is not grown in Nova Scotia, and enjoy it! Fruits contain a large number of naturally occurring vitamins, minerals and phytochemicals that promote health. Its low sodium content makes it beneficial in losing weight, as there is no water retention. Its high fiber content gives us energy and fills us up so that we don't feel hungry. Antioxidants in fruit reduce the risk of cardiovascular disease and some cancers. Fruit can also lower blood pressure and cholesterol and slow down the aging process.

Sometimes we get caught-up in the glycemic index in our choice of fruits, but when we consume whole plant foods we are less likely to feel hungry. We also benefit from this unprocessed fibre-rich food with all of its live enzymes intact. One fruit, roughly the size of a tennis ball, is the equivalent of 1/2 cup of juice. But choose the whole fruit for its fiber, as fruit juice is naturally high in sugar, can reap havoc with our blood sugar and lead to Candida. The Raw Live Vegan menu planners make it easy to use up the 15%. My whole fruit consumption is gone at breakfast.

The avocado is a high fat fruit that is commonly considered a vegetable. Avocados are a complete source of protein and contain all the essential amino acids. Their buttery flesh contains high amounts of monounsaturated fat, known as oleic acid, which lowers cholesterol by decreasing LDL (the bad cholesterol which clogs arteries) and increasing HDL (the good cholesterol which facilitates the transport of cholesterol in the blood and reduces the risk of coronary heart disease and atherosclerosis). Avocados are a rich source of vitamin E, which aids in the formation of red blood cells, and vitamin C, which helps prevent cardiovascular disease. Both vitamin C and E are known for their antioxidants, which protect cells and tissue from the damaging effects of free radicals. Avocados also contain vitamin K, which is essential for blood coagulation, bone density and calcium absorption. Folate, which aids in the development of tissues and cells, is another important vitamin found in avocados.

Avocados are also rich in minerals. They contain potassium, calcium, phosphorus, zinc and selenium. Potassium maintains the electrolyte balance in the body, regulates blood pressure, and lowers the risk of heart disease and stroke.

Calcium and phosphorus are essential for growth of strong bones and teeth. Zinc facilitates the proper functioning of the immune system, energy metabolism and digestion. Despite being rich in fats, the avocado can help you lose weight, due to its high concentration of health promoting monounsaturated fatty acids. The avocado is very alkaline and will contribute to your overall wellbeing. Check out where it lies on the pH chart. The avocado could easily switch places with the apple. In fact, the jingle, "an apple a day..." could better be stated, "an avocado a day keeps the doctor away!"

Vegetables

Vegetables and sea vegetables should make up 60% of our daily food intake.

Vegetables and sea vegetables should make up 60% of our daily food intake. Fresh vegetables of all kinds, starchy, non-starchy and leafy green can be enjoyed at any time - the darker the better. Vegetables provide the body with needed vitamins, minerals and fibre. When we buy organic we get more than our money's worth in vitamin and mineral content. Most commercially grown vegetables are nutrient and vitamin depleted due to the chemical sprays and dyes that are used to make them picture perfect, appealing to our visual senses.

As all vegetables from every color of the rainbow provide different and necessary vitamins and nutrients to our daily nutrition and wellbeing, they are unlimited on this program. Brassica a genus of the Cruciferous vegetables including broccoli, cauliflower, collard greens and cabbage are famously healthy and cancer-fighting vegetables. Dark green vegetables are the most beneficial, so try to consume 3 cups a day. Watercress, cabbage, spinach and kale contain carotenoids that protect, delay and may prevent the onset of degenerative age-related eye diseases such as cataracts or macular degeneration. Dark green leafy vegetables also contain vitamins C and E, both powerful antioxidants that boost our immune system to help it fight mutating cancerous cells and heart disease. Dark green vegetables also contain the iron, which we formerly got from red meat. Red, orange and yellow colored fruits and vegetables such as melon, tomatoes, carrots, and apricots contain vitamins A, C and E. All of these vitamins help fight certain types of cancer by neutralizing free radicals in the body.

Greens Plus and Spirulina provide other means of getting important vitamins and minerals through vegetables. *Greens Plus* is a concentrated vegetable powder found at health food stores, in the health food section of the local grocery store or online. Spirulina is blue-green algae containing trace amounts of vitamins, minerals and amino acids plus the important fatty acids our body needs every day. I use Spirulina and *Greens Plus* in a blender with water, fruit and protein powder, to make a tasty, healthy morning shake. When choosing protein powders for our morning shakes, it is important to remember that not all protein powders are created equal. In fact, whey and soy-based protein powders are highly acidic and difficult for our body to process. Also, the high temperature and chemicals used to remove fat and carbohydrates and create a protein isolate leave behind toxic residues. Acid-based proteins such as whey and soy cause inflammation, the last thing we need when trying to lead an active lifestyle! Instead, try the "Vega" brand complete whole Food Health Optimizer, all-in-one, natural plant-based formula. It contains 100% RDI (recommended daily intake) of vitamins and minerals per serving, is rich in protein, fibre, omega-3 EFAs (essential fatty acids), antioxidants and phytonutrients. It contains no common allergens, is alkaline-forming and easy to digest. Plant-based proteins protect against chronic diseases, are low in saturated fat and promote overall health. So look for plant-based proteins such as hemp, spirulina, raw alfalfa juice, green pea protein, and raw sprouted rice as choices in plant-based protein powders. The protein shake is best consumed after a workout.

Wheatgrass juice contains most of the vitamins and minerals needed to sustain life. It also contains calcium, iron, magnesium, phosphorus, potassium, sodium, sulphur, cobalt and zinc. Two ounces of wheat grass juice is to equal to three pounds of organic vegetables in vitamin and mineral equivalency. Its chlorophyll removes toxins from our cells and fatty tissues, helps replenish red blood cells and reduces anemia. Studies have shown that after five short days on wheat grass the red blood cell count returns to normal. We all know chlorophyll is great for breath as it neutralizes odor. For those of us that have town water treated with fluoride it is nice to know that one ounce of wheatgrass can neutralize one gallon of fluoridated water by converting the fluorine into harmless calcium phosphate. Now that is better for your teeth! Mix this juice in with your bath water to get rid of sores, itching and pimples. Use a tincture in a pot of water to clean vegetables and fruit that may have come in contact with harmful chemicals. Chlorophyll is also known to clear up congestion and head colds within 24 hours.

Wheatgrass helps stop the growth and development of unfriendly bacteria by creating an unfriendly environment. It is high in beta-carotene, which can contribute to a reduction in the development of certain cancers. The wheat berry is stored energy which, when converted to simpler sugars, is a quick source of energy. Start by drinking only one ounce a day. You will be amazed how much grass is required to make one ounce of wheatgrass juice! CAUTION HERE: wheatgrass is powerful, as its reaction against toxins is immediate. This leaves mucus in our stomach, which can cause nausea, so less is more. When sprouting wheatgrass, harvest and drink it on the same day.

Sea Vegetables

Sea vegetables are a great addition to the diet and are ready to eat in nori, kelp, dulse, arame, wakami and hijiki. They contain cobalt, zinc, iron, chlorine, manganese, magnesium and nickel. Try sprinkling some dried seaweed on a salad. Sea vegetables are also high in iodine, which only comes from the sea. The thyroid needs iodine to manufacture thyroxin, which aids the metabolic rate of digestion. Without enough thyroxin, food is digested too slowly and is stored as fat. According to The World Health Organization (*The Lancet*, July 2008), the brain requires iodine to function. Iodine deficiency is linked to mental retardation. It is also a contributing factor to enlarged adenoids, goiter, fatigue, colds and infections.

Whole Grains

The next three food groups combine to make up approximately 15% of the daily food intake (whole grains, nuts & seeds and Legumes).

The next three food groups, combined, make up 15% of the daily food intake. They include whole grains, nuts and seeds. Whole grains in the Raw Live Vegan program include: barley, buckwheat, kamut, quinoa, rye, spelt, steel oats, wheat and wild rice. Whole grain foods are a natural source of vitamins A, E and B6. They also contain the minerals selenium, zinc, copper and iron, and supply both soluble and insoluble fibre. Soluble fibre helps reduce blood cholesterol. Insoluble fibre helps maintain gastrointestinal and bowel health. Whole grains are also an excellent source of complex carbohydrates. Carbohydrates get a bad reputation, as we confuse refined carbohydrates (the bad ones) with unrefined (complex) carbohydrates, which are present in whole plant foods. Multigrain is never to be confused with 'whole grain.' Whole grains must be soaked in twice the amount of water for about 12 hours and rinsed well before they are ready to eat.

It is also important to distinguish between intact and refined whole grains. Intact whole grains still retain their germ and bran components, which contribute important nutrients and fibre to the diet. Refined grains lose the germ and bran during the milling process. Intact whole grains include: buckwheat groats, kamut, oat groats, quinoa, rye, ground flax, barley and wild rice.

Fibre is a unique category of carbohydrate because it does not breakdown in our digestive tract, but passes through unabsorbed. The skins and seeds of whole grains contain plenty of fibre, which our body needs to help cleanse and rid itself of waste and toxins. Fibre keeps bowel movements regular, which lowers our risk of constipation, diverticulitis and bowel cancer. It also lowers our cholesterol, which keeps our heart healthy. Stores will market colon cleansers, but I am here to tell you that if you change your eating to raw, constipation will be a thing of the past. The best colon cleanser is flax.

There is plenty of fibre built into this program. We get 1 tablespoon of ground flax in our morning *Greens Plus* shake. We get flax seeds and ground flax in our crackers and breakfast bread. We also get fibre in our fruits, vegetables, beans, nuts and seeds. Our intestine contains more than 300 different types of bacteria - some good, some bad. The good bacteria will flourish and aid your immune system when you increase your intake of raw plant food. The opposite happens when food intake from refined sugars supports the microorganisms that promote disease.

Nuts & Seeds

Raw nuts of all kinds are an important component of this program. They include almonds, Brazil nuts, coconuts, filberts, macadamia nuts, hazelnuts, pecans, pine nuts and walnuts, to name a few. Keep in mind that peanuts and cashews contain oil that is difficult to digest. Also, raw nuts must be soaked before they are eaten (see soaking chart for instructions). Nuts, unlike grains, contain an enzyme inhibitor that prevents them from sprouting prematurely. This inhibitor also plays havoc on our GI tract as it creates discomfort during digestion. Soaking our nuts in one tablespoon of salt per liter of water activates the enzymes that remove the enzyme inhibitors and allows us to digest them properly. Choose the type of nut you use the most in your favorite recipes. Soak them in the salt and water overnight, drain and refill the jar with water to continue soaking. Store them in the refrigerator ready for use and be sure to change the water daily. I add a tablespoon of walnuts, which are a great source of Omega-3, to my morning cereal, so I keep a mason jar of walnuts, topped up with water, in my refrigerator. My husband and I go through this in about four days. When they are done, I know it is time to soak more nuts and grains for breakfast.

Raw seeds on the program include: alfalfa, caraway, clover, fenugreek, flax, pumpkin, radish, red clover, sesame, sunflower, wheatgrass and hemp seeds. Some seeds are great for salad toppings for extra fiber. Some are good soaked and sprouted. The shelf life of seeds can be doubled through refrigeration and increased four to five times more by freezing them. Some seeds are meant to be consumed immediately after sprouting, such as alfalfa, broccoli and wheatgrass. Others are meant to be planted in soil or grown hydroponically after they are sprouted, such as sunflower or wheat grass seeds. Wheat grass can be grown without soil on a special germination seedling flat, which has many holes to support soil-free growing and can be used over and over. We just spray the seeds with water and watch them grow.

The varieties of nuts and seeds available on the market are endless. I buy seeds I can't find locally on line. My health food store and supermarket are excellent sources too. I also buy in bulk and freeze. Be careful not by buy blanched, spiced or sweetened nuts or seeds. You need to know that they are "raw."

Legumes

Legumes are a high quality protein enjoyed by several cultures worldwide. They include: adzuki beans, anasazi beans, black beans, black-eyed peas, chickpeas, endamame beans, mung beans, northern white beans, pinto beans, fava beans, lentils, lima beans, peas, and red kidney beans. Legumes offer amazing health benefits. Their complex carbohydrates provide energy to the brain for clear thinking, and to the muscles to get us through the demands of the day. They are an excellent source of vitamins, zinc, calcium, iron, magnesium, folic acid, copper, protein, fibre, and amino acids that can prevent heart disease and cancer. As they are high in soluble fiber and low in fat they are superior to animal protein. Soluble fiber prevents fluctuations in blood sugar, thereby providing the body with a stable level of sugar that is used for energy and not stored as fat. Soluble fiber helps with regularity. It can also cause flatulence, but this decreases as our body gets used to digesting them more regularly. As they have a low glycemic index and prevent a sharp rise in blood sugar, they are of great benefit to diabetics, hypoglycemics and to those who are insulin resistant.

Legumes combat the damage LDL (bad cholesterol) causes to our blood, thereby reducing the risk of heart disease. They also slow down the absorption of carbohydrates. Due to their folic acid content, which protects fetuses from developing spina bifida, they are beneficial to pregnant women. A big bonus is that the flavonoids in legumes can act as the female hormone estrogen. Phytoestrogens are estrogen-like products derived from plants. Although they are not the same as the hormones found in the female body, they have a beneficial effect. Phytoestrogens bind to estrogen receptors. When they bind they exert a balancing effect. This means that if your estrogen is low they will have an estrogenic effect that raises estrogen levels to a point where they reduce the incidence of hot flashes. If the estrogen is too high, they will block estrogen production in a similar manner as treatment for PMS. Phytoestrogens do not stimulate the growth of estrogen. In fact, studies have shown that they can inhibit the growth of breast tumours in animals.

As legumes offer incredible benefits to human health, a few tablespoons at each meal are encouraged. I buy in bulk and freeze them for longer storage. Sprouting legumes and seeds offers a great source of protein, high fibre and vitamins C, B-complex and A, without the fat and cholesterol. In the sprouting process, starches are converted to simple sugars, making them easy to digest. What else will grow in any climate, will rival meat in nutritive value, will mature in 3 to 5 days, may be planted any day of the year, requires neither soil nor sun, will produce more nutritional vitamin C than tomatoes and can be eaten raw?

Fats & Oils

The next three groups should take up 10% of your daily intake (*Fats, Oils & Sweeteners*).

The next three groups should comprise 10% of our daily intake. They include fats, oils and sweeteners. Fats are essential to optimal health. Raw plant foods are rich in essential fatty acids. Fats and oils on the Raw Live Vegan program include: coconut oil, flax oil, grape-seed oil, hemp oil, organic cold-pressed extra virgin olive oil, stone ground olive oil, walnut oil, avocados and sunflower oil. Oils containing omega-6 fatty acids include safflower oil, wheat germ oil, walnut oil, sesame oil and olive oil. Omega-3 fatty acids are found in butternuts, chia seeds, flaxseeds, flaxseed oil, hempseed and hempseed oil and walnuts. Flaxseeds must be ground to be absorbed. Leafy greens such as kale, lettuce and spinach are also excellent sources of Omega-3.

The old way of thinking said that one had to eliminate cholesterol to lose weight. Today we know there is good cholesterol and bad cholesterol and the role each plays in our health. As cholesterol cannot dissolve in the blood, carriers must transport it to and from cells. These carriers are found in cholesterol and are called lipoproteins. Low-density lipoprotein or LDL is also known as bad cholesterol. This is the kind of cholesterol that circulates in blood and combines with other substances to form plaque on the inner walls of arteries that feed to the heart and brain. Plaque narrows the arteries and obstructs blood flow. When a clot forms and blocks the narrowed artery, heart attack or stroke can occur. High-density lipoprotein or HDL is known as good cholesterol, because it is thought to carry cholesterol away from the arteries to the liver, where it is processed and eliminated. In this way HDL is thought to protect us from heart attack or stroke. HDL leaves us feeling satisfied as it slows down and regulates the rate at which glucose enters the blood stream, making it slow and controlled. It also aids mental comprehension, provides a protective covering to our organ tissues and facilitates healthy nerve conduction. We need cholesterol for cell replication. Cholesterol is also important to a whole class of hormones known as steroid hormones critical to life. These hormones determine our sexuality, control our reproductive process, and regulate blood sugar levels and mineral metabolism.

Recommended oils are flax seed oil, hemp seed oil, cold pressed olive oil, sesame oil, sunflower oil and coconut oil. Non-hydrogenated low fat spreads include organic sunflower butter and almond butter, they are great flavour boosters and high quality spreads for use in dips or oils for flavourings and are used in many raw live vegan recipes. They can add to sauces on vegetables and are just plain delicious on our multigrain breads. It is best to serve fats in dressings for salads or in marinades or spreads. Oils should be stored in the refrigerator after purchasing.

Sweeteners

Sweeteners on the Raw Live Vegan program include: Lakanto, dates, yacon syrup, agave syrup, cane juice, coconut sugar, sucanat, maple syrup, stevia, and xylitol. Lakanto is an all-natural sweetener that looks and tastes like sugar and has a zero glycemic index. Lakanto comes from combined Erythritol (fermented erythritol is a corn alcohol) and Luo Han Guo extract, a fruit found in the Guilin Mountains in southern China. The reason erythritol is combined with the Chinese fruit Luo Han Guo is due to the fruit extract being 300 times sweeter than sugar so it is difficult to use. Since mouth bacteria can't metabolize Lakanto, it's kid-friendly too and won't cause cavities or contribute to tooth decay.

Lakanto is expensive, but like anything in life we have to prioritize the benefit of each product according to our own clinical diagnosis. Another point of interest is that the Luo Han Guo fruit acts as an anti-carcinogenic as well as an anti-inflammatory and antioxidant, and it is beneficial in treating certain digestive ailments. Like anything, I always recommend listing products and supplements that you consume to share with your doctor in case of a natural substance interacts negatively with a prescribed medication. Yacon syrup is another favourite due to its benefits to the GI tract. (Yes, we have found a sweetener that will actually benefit our GI tract). The yacon plant, Smallanthus sonchifolius, is indigenous to the high altitudes of the Andes Mountains, in Peru. Yacon tastes similar to jicama, but is biologically closer to the sunflower family. It is often compared to molasses, caramel or honey in taste. Yacon root contains a special type of sugar known as oligofructose, or fructo-oligosaccharide (FOS). The syrup contains up to 50% FOS. Because the human body has no enzyme to hydrolyze (process) FOS, it passes through the system without leaving behind absorbable sugar compounds. This means that it is not converted to glucose in the bloodstream and passes through the digestive tract unmetabolized. As it is not processed in the body, it is generally referred to as 'sugar free.' Yacon also is relatively low in calories, compared to most other sweeteners. As the process to create it is vegan, vegans who are averse to refined sugar can use it. Try swirling yacon syrup in your breakfast cereal, spread it over fruit, or use it to sweeten tea. Caution here: the sweetness is strong so less is more.

Some studies have suggested that yacon syrup may be beneficial to the body in moderate amounts. It contains and promotes healthy bacteria that aid in cleaning the colon and regulating the digestive system. These un-metabolized sugars then become food for the friendly bacteria that live in the colon, increasing their population and simultaneously decreasing harmful bacteria. When something has this effect on our intestinal flora it is known as 'prebiotic' and is beneficial for overall colon health. It regulates intestinal flora, which reduces constipation, improves absorption of calcium, magnesium and other vitamins, reduces cholesterol and triglyceride levels and boosts the immune system.

In Peru, the leaves of the yacon plant are eaten for its nutritional properties. In Brazil, the leaves are brewed into a tea to fight diabetes. In Bolivia, diabetics and people suffering from digestive and renal disorders eat them to improve health.

Many health food experts consider yacon syrup to be a newly discovered wonder food. Further studies must be conducted to determine its beneficial health effects. And as any insulin-derived sweetener has large amounts of fructose, the same concerns over the health effects of fructose in yacon syrup apply.

In closing this section on Allowable Foods, it is prudent to remember fruits and vegetables make up the largest part of our daily intake so take the time to shop your local markets, marvel at the variety and be tempted to try something different, something new and make it tasty!

Diets rich in fruit and vegetables can prevent a number of serious illnesses such as cancer, high blood pressure and cardiovascular disease. We all see the burden on our health care system caused by diets based on processed convenience foods. Our current poor health is a boon to the pharmaceutical industry. The list of nasty ingredients in convenience foods is long. But what is in our fruits and vegetables? They are made up of water and essential vitamins and minerals that are lacking in most processed foods. With the abundance of fruit and vegetables available to us, it is not difficult to consume the recommended 9 servings per day, especially if you are introducing them into your morning shake, or your marinades, dips, and other beverages. A medium sized fruit or 1/2 cup is a single serving. One cup of vegetables is a vegetable serving. Three tablespoons of pulses - chickpeas, beans, lentils or sprouts - is a serving. Remember raw is better, as cooking destroys the vitamin C and other water-soluble nutrients found in these nutritious foods. Remember to wash fruit and vegetables thoroughly to remove dirt and insects; do not leave in water to soak, as they will lose their vitamins and minerals to the water. I use a vinegar soak with water and rub the skins well before drying them and storing them in the refrigerator.

Allowable Foods Lists

Fruit

Apples	Grapefruit	Pineapple
Avocados	Figs	Plums
Apricots	Mangoes	Prunes
Bananas	Melons	Raisins
Berries	Oranges	Tomatoes
Cantaloupe	Papaya	
Currants	Peaches	
Dates	Pears	

Nuts & Seeds

Almonds	Hazelnuts	Sesame Tahini
Brazil Nuts	Pine Nuts	Sunflower Seeds
Cashews	Pistachio Nuts	Walnuts
Chia Seeds	Psyllium seeds	
Flax Seeds	Poppy Seeds	

Vinegars & Miscellaneous

Apple Cider	*Greens Plus* Pdr	Probiotic Pdr
Red Wine	Miso Light	Nama Shoyu
White Wine	Miso Dark	Nut Butters
Tahini	Tamari	Spirulina Pdr

Beans / Oils / Seeds

Beans	Oils	Seeds
Adzuki	Flax Seed Oil	Alfalfa
Lentils	Hemp Seed Oil	Broccoli
Mung	Olive Oil	Radishes

Vegetables

Asparagus	Kale	Peppers
Beans	Garlic	Radishes
Carrots	Lettuce	Sweet Potato
Cauliflower	Mushrooms	Turnips
Celery	Olives	Yams
Corn	Onions	Zucchini
Dandelion	Parsnips	
Eggplant	Peas	

Grains

Amaranth	Pdr	Rye
Barley	Kamut	Red Hard
Buckwheat	Millet	Wheat
Ground Flax	Quinoa	Wild Rice

Sea Products

Dulse	Nori Wraps	Sea Vegetables
Kelp	Sea Noodles	Wakami

Flavoring

Almond	Cocoa	Pure Vanilla
Cacao	Orange Oil	Vanilla Beans

Protein Sources on the Raw Live Vegan Diet

One of the biggest food falsehoods that I know of is the animal protein delusion. We are lead to believe that all of our protein must come from animal food sources when, in fact, there are a variety of healthier plant-based proteins. The following chart shows nutrient values for both plant and animal proteins. This should reassure you that plant proteins are a safer and healthier dietary option.

Nutrient Comparison: Plant Vs. Animal

The World Health Organization recommends that 2-10% of daily calories come from protein sources; remember plants are also protein sources. T. Colin Campbell's study, "The China Study" found that most westerners consume somewhere between 120 - 158% more animal-based protein than recommended. North Americans are the sickest population on the planet, with exploding rates of obesity, Type II Diabetes and heart disease. The healthiest populations are those that derive their food from plants. The recommended protein intake is .08 grams of protein for each kilogram of body weight. For example: a 150lb person in kilograms weighs 68kg. Multiplying 68kg times .08, equals 55 grams of protein per day. If you are consuming plant-based protein, you could get 21 grams of protein from your cereal of buckwheat muesli and at least 15 grams of protein from your breakfast shake. An additional 15 grams of protein could come from your salad or vegetable entrees at lunch and dinner. So, you can easily exceed the recommended daily intake of protein based on plant-based protein but then again you are also getting more than the required daily intake of fruits and vegetables as a bonus! Each gram of protein provides 4 calories. To get 50 grams of protein on a 2,000 calorie per day diet, just 10% of your calories come from plant-based proteins. This is not hard to do. On the Raw Live Vegan program your protein needs will never be lacking!

Nutrient Comparison: Plant Vs. Animal

Nutrient	Plant Source	Animal Source
Cholesterol per (mg)	0	137
Fat (g)	4	36
Protein (g)	33	34
Beta-carotene (mcg)	29,919	17
Dietary Fiber (g)	31	0
Vitamin C (mg)	293	4
Folate (mcg)	1168	19
Vitamin E (mg)	20	2
Magnesium (mg)	548	51
Calcium (mg)	545	252

Fibre Essential to Health

Fibre is only found in plants – welcome to your new healthy lifestyle of raw live vegan! There is no fibre found in animal meat. There are two types of Fibre: Soluble fibre and Insoluble fibre.

Soluble Fibre is food that will begin to dissolve and form a gel in water. Soluble fibre has been shown to lower cholesterol, protecting the heart from disease. Soluble fibre slows down the absorption of glucose into the bloodstream, helping to prevent diabetes and obesity. Soluble fibre can be found in oats, legumes, brown rice barley, fruits (especially apples), and some green vegetables like broccoli. Soluble fibre is very satisfying, leaving you feeling full on less food and better able to control weight.

Insoluble Fibre will pass through the digestive system without being digested. This type of fibre adds bulk to the stool, making it easier and faster to pass through the digestive system. Insoluble Fibre can be found in whole grains, wheat bran, the skins of many fruits and vegetables, seeds, nuts and dried beans.

Fibre is especially important for older persons as their digestive system slows down with aging. On the raw live vegan lifestyle you will experience increased painless bowel movements. By increased consumption of fibre you avoid constipation, diverticulitis (small hernias of the bowel tract) and reduce the risk of colon cancer. Foods on the raw live vegan plan are high in hydration since they are not cooked; allowing consumption of fibre to be more easily managed than for those that eat an animal based diet. Retail stores will market stool softeners, enemas, and my favourite, fibre in a container! I trust Mother Nature and her healing bounty of organic fruits and vegetables and whole grains, nuts and seeds before I would ever trust anything chemical! If you change your eating to raw, constipation will be a thing of the past. The best colon cleanser is flax! Flax starts at point of entry, the mouth, and doesn't stop doing its' intended job until it exits into the toilet! On this program you will be getting 1 tablespoon of ground flax in your morning *Greens Plus* shake, you will get flax seeds, and ground flax in crackers and in bread, plus the natural roughage from raw fruits and vegetables eaten the way nature intended, there is plenty of fibre built in to this program. Your intestine contains more than 300 different types of bacteria some good, some bad, the good will flourish and aid your immune system when you increase your intake of raw plant food. The opposite happens when food intake from refined sugars supports the microorganisms that promote disease.

You will find many charts rating foods and their fibre content; you will see that many differ. Some offer fibre content on cooked, dried and raw fibre. You will see that cooked has more fibre than raw, while dried more than cooked or raw. Remember raw has higher water content – a very important combination with its' fibre component. With the mini list provided, you will see with just some of the foods enjoyed on our raw live vegan plan you will more than achieve the recommended daily amount of fibre, where most other plans fail miserably!

When it comes to fibre content, estimates vary from one source to the next, as do calories. Also, take into consideration the fact that the estimates also vary between raw, dried and cooked foods. You will not see the fibre count for a cooked vegetable, even though it would be above 1 gram, since this chart deals with the raw live vegan plan. Also note that when food is dried, the grams per portion are less due to no water content. Juices are left off, as their fibre content depends on if the manufacturer includes pulp or not. The counts are close estimates. This chart shows the higher food choices containing 1 gram of fibre or more. We need 25-40 grams of fibre a day.

* It is important to take psyllium seed with plenty of water to avoid risk of choking. Since the herb is a fiber, taking it without at least eight ounces of water can cause the fibrous herb to swell up in the esophagus or throat. Suggested serving size is one teaspoon of psyllium seeds with 8 oz. of water, three times a day to treat constipation.

Grams of Fibre in Our Food

Fruit/Portion - Fibre (g)

Food	Fibre (g)
Apple, raw with skin, 1 medium	4.0
Apple, dried, 10 rings	5.6
Apricot, raw with skin, 3 "small"	3.1
Apricots, dried, 5 pieces	2.9
Avocado raw, 1/2 cup 125 mL	3.0
Banana, raw, 1 "medium"	3.0
Blackberries, raw, 1/2 cup/125 mL	4.0
Cantaloupe, 1/4 of melon	1.3
Cherries, raw, 10 pieces/30mL	1.7
Cranberries, raw dried, 1/2 cup/125 mL	5.7
Currants, black, 6 tablespoons, 90 mL	8.5
Currants, dried, 1 tablespoon, 15 mL	6.5
Currants, red 6 tablespoons, 90 mL	8.0
Dates, dried, 2 pieces	1.2
Figs, raw, 3 pieces	5.0
Figs dried	5.2
Grapes, white, raw, 1/2 cup, 125 mL	1.0
Kiwi, 1 medium	2.1
Lemon, raw, 1 tablespoon, 15 mL	5.0
Lettuce leaves, 4 leaves	1.6
Loganberries, raw, 1/2 cup, 125 mL	6.0
Mangoes, raw, 1/2 cup/125 mL	1.5
Nectarines, raw, 1/2 cup/125 mL	2.0
Olives in brine, 5 pieces	3.5
Orange, whole, raw, 1 "medium"	3.0
Papaya, 1 "medium"	5.5
Passion fruit, whole, raw, 1/2 cup/125 mL	12.0
Passion fruit, dried, 2 tablespoons, 30 mL	14.5
Peach, raw, 1 "medium"	1.4
Peach, dried, 5 pieces	5.3
Pear, raw, 1 "medium"	5.08
Pear, dried, 5 pieces	11.5
Pineapple, raw, 1/3 cup/80 mL	1.0
Plums, 1/2 cup/ 125 mL	4.0
Pomegranate, 1/2 "medium"	2.8
Prunes, raw, 5 prunes	4.0
Quince, raw, 1/2 cup/125 mL	6.5
Raisins, dried, 1/4 cup/60 mL	3.1
Raspberries, raw, 1/2 cup/125 mL	4.0
Strawberries, 1/2 cup/125 mL	2.0
Tangerine, 1 "medium"	1.5

Nuts/Portion - Fibre (g)

Almonds, raw, 10 nuts	1.1
Brazil nuts, raw, 5 nuts	2.1
Cashews, 2 tablespoons/30 mL	1.0
Chestnuts, raw 4 nuts	7.0
Coconut, dried, 1 tablespoon/15 mL	3.4
Hazelnuts, raw, 10 nuts	6.0
Peanuts, raw, 2 tablespoons/30 mL	5.5
Walnuts, raw, 5 nuts	5.0
Miscellaneous nuts, 1/4 cup/30mL	2.0-4.0

Vegetable/ Portion - Fibre (g)

Broccoli, raw, 1/2 cup 125 mL	3.8
Cabbage, raw, 1/2 cup/125 mL	1.5
Carrots, raw, 1/2 cup/125 mL	3.4
Cauliflower, raw, 1/2 cup/125 mL	4.0
Celery, raw, 1/2 cup/125 mL	4.0
Mushrooms, raw, 2 tablespoons, 30 mL	2.5
Onions, raw, 1 tablespoon, 15 mL	1.5
Parsley, raw, 4 tablespoons/60 mL	1.2
Peppers, raw, 1 cup, 250 mL	2.4
Pumpkin, raw, 1/2 cup/125 mL	2.0
Radishes, raw, 1/4 cup/60 mL	3.0
Sauerkraut, 2/3 cup/160 mL	3.1
Tomato, raw, 1/2 cup 125 mL	1.5

Bean Sprouts/ Portion - Fibre (g)

Adzuki beans, 1/2 cup/125 mL	7.0
Chickpeas, 1/2 cup/125 mL	7.0
Lentils, 1/2 cup/125 mL	7.0
Mung, 1/2 cup/125 mL	7.0

Grains/ Portion - Fibre (g)

Amaranth, raw, soaked, 1/2 cup/125 mL	15.2
Barley, pearled, raw, soaked, 1/2 cup/125 mL	7.0
Bran, raw oat bran, 1/2 cup/125 mL	6.6
Buckwheat, raw, soaked, 1/2 cup/125 mL	8.0
Kamut, raw, soaked, 1/4 cup/60 mL	5.0
Millet, raw soaked, 1/2 cup/125 mL	3.6
Oat groats, raw, soaked, 1/2 cup/125 mL	2.0
Wild rice, raw soaked, 1 cup/250 mL	10.0
Quinoa, raw soaked, 1/4 cup/60 mL	2.5

Seeds/ Portion - Fibre (g)
Flax seeds, ground, 2 tablespoons, 30 mL	6.6
*Psyllium, seeds, 2 tablespoons/30 mL	18.0
Pumpkin seeds, raw, 1/4 cup/60 mL	4.12
Sunflower seeds, raw, 2 tablespoons/30 mL	1.0
Sesame seeds, raw, 2 1/2 tablespoons/45 mL	1.0

Eat To Live!

Our grandparents enjoyed the secret to a long life. They found it in the nutritious, wholesome, unprocessed foods they ate. Oftentimes, they grew it themselves. Somehow, we have moved away from this healthy lifestyle, into one that is fast-paced and competitive. In the process, we have embraced a diet that has conformed to it, all in the name of convenience. We often eat on the fly, rarely taking the time to prepare a nutritious, well-balanced meal to share with our families around the dinner table. Instead, we choose processed foods that we pop into the oven or the microwave, or worse – pick up at the drive-through of a fast food outlet. Despite all of this, we consider ourselves to be healthy, at least by today's standards. Yet the typical North American diet can lead to high cholesterol, diabetes, heart disease, and cancer.

Food is a powerful tool. It has the ability to make us sick or to cure us. Even in today's busy world, we shall be conscious of the importance of nutritious food and of the way we prepare it. A healthy menu includes fruits, vegetables, fibre, protein and hydration on a daily basis. Include Superfoods, as they aid health and are nutrient dense, antioxidant rich, disease fighting, anti-aging and, yes, beautifying. They also enhance wellbeing and boost the immune system. Superfoods include beans, blueberries, broccoli, oats, oranges, pumpkin, soy, spinach, tea, tomatoes, flax seeds, almonds and walnuts, to name a few; and they are all conveniently available at your local supermarket. Choose dark greens, deep reds and vibrant yellows, and build your rainbow from a variety of unprocessed, organic fruits and vegetables. Be sure to reward yourself with a little chocolate that contains at least 60% cocoa, before checking out.

Eat mindfully. Read the ingredients on packaged food before putting it into your grocery cart. You will find that most packaged foods contain a list of ingredients a mile long. If you don't know what something is and can't even pronounce it, are you sure you want to feed it to your family? Fresh fruits and vegetables, beans, nuts and seeds don't come with a list, as they include a single, natural ingredient; they are what you see. Countless books have been written about the benefits of unrefined wholesome foods in their purest state and how they aid health and wellbeing. But I have yet to read a single book on the benefits of processed foods. So why is it hard to accept the raw live vegan as anything other then healthy! Foods that are genetically modified fill our grocery shops and consumers fill their carts without a blink of an eye; how have we allowed ourselves to come to this?

The processed food industry continually bombards us with commercials on fast, fun, must-have foods. According to the media, we live to eat, when, in fact, we shall eat to live. Commercials, in print and broadcast media, encourage us to eat just about anywhere: at mealtime; at work; when out with friends; while watching television; or driving in the car. They have even suggested that we can eat in our sleep. We have all seen the commercial of the sleepwalker, mindlessly entering the kitchen, in the dead of night, opening the refrigerator and sticking his head in. In short, according to the media, food has no down time. On the contrary, our body needs a break from food, as it needs time to digest. This means nothing going into the gut, while the body does its job digesting food that passes through the GI tract. But, if we follow the advice we see on TV, we will put our systems into overdrive. It's much better to turn it off, and get outside to enjoy some activity.

The foods we use in the Raw Live Vegan program help to trim and revitalize the body. We too must be mindful to eat consciously to the point of being satisfied, not full. If we eat until we are full and cannot eat anymore, then we have eaten too much. If we eat until satisfied and wait 20 minutes to see if we want to finish what is on our plate you will be astonished that you will find you are full! The foods on the raw live vegan plan are not preserved, processed, pasteurized, adulterated or irradiated. They are not baked, boiled, braised, barbequed or microwaved. Most of our recipes focus on the raw aspect of food preparation. Raw foods contain enzymes that aid in digestion and are readily absorbed into the bloodstream. Looking back into the history of food, we find that traditional meals, in many cultures, opened with a salad, as the fresh, raw, live aspect of this dish aided in the digestion of courses that followed.

Raw food affects your body's chemistry. The majority of raw foods are alkaline, as opposed to acidic, which is very important for pH balance. Acidic, chemically laden, high fat, high sugar, cooked or processed foods can lead to inflammatory diseases, such as rheumatoid arthritis and osteoarthritis. This occurs when the body takes alkalizing minerals from bone to correct the body's pH balance. Raw food may not cure all aliments, but it will do far more for your body than a high fat, high sugar, acidic diet. And it is never cooked at temperatures above 118 degrees Fahrenheit. Temperatures above this kill the natural enzymes that boost your body's immune system and help it fight off disease.

Being conscious of what you eat lends to being observant of those around you and the dietary choices they make. This is a time for silent observation, and not for critiquing. We may see others order high-fat, high sugar foods from a menu; all the while remarking on how tired they feel or how much weight they have gained. They may even venture into the topic of family genetics, where a history of diabetes or heart disease is well documented. And they may complain of having no time to address any of these issues, in their busy lives, as they excuse themselves from the table to go outside for a cigarette! The diplomatic thing to do is to hold your tongue. You would be mistaken if you thought that they didn't know the difference between your healthy choices and their bad ones. Perhaps they are dealing with problems in their personal lives that you are not aware of. Or maybe they are simply not ready to make a change. This is not the time or place to engage in a public banter about diet and lifestyle. Instead, wait until they ask you, directly, what it is that you do to maintain your youthful vitality. Then, you could suggest getting together, over a nice cup of green tea, to discuss this very subject. If they are really interested, they will eagerly accept your invitation and investigate your suggestions further. If they are not, it may simply be their way complimenting you. But, perhaps some time in the future, they will be interested in discussing strategies for attaining optimal health. The trick is to offer them an open-ended invitation that they can follow-up on when they are ready.

Mindful eaters who enjoy RAW Live Vegan Food, are not all 100% RAW Foodies. But, all will affirm that the more RAW the better, simply because when you cook it, you cook out the vitamins and nutrients. If it is heat you want, get it through spices, or warm it up to 118 degrees Fahrenheit. Going 80% RAW Live Vegan is a realistic goal. This site will cover the varying aspects of the Raw Live Vegan lifestyle, in years to come. If you have just started the program, you are on the right path. Check into our website often; read our new articles, try our new recipes, and continue to reap the rewards gained by eating raw food.

Grocery List

FRUIT

- Apples
- Apricots
- Bananas
- Berries
- Cantaloupe
- Coconut
- Currants
- Dates
- Figs
- Grapefruit
- Honeydew melon
- Kiwi
- Mango
- Oranges
- Papaya
- Peaches
- Pears
- Pineapple
- Plums
- Prunes
- Raisins, grapes
- Watermelon

VEGETABLES

- Asparagus
- Fresh basil
- Snap beans
- Carrots
- Cauliflower
- Celery
- Cilantro
- Corn
- Cucumber
- Dandelion greens
- Eggplant
- Garlic cloves
- Green giant juice
- Horseradish
- Kale
- Kelp
- Leeks
- Onions
- Parsley
- Peas
- Peppers
- Radishes
- Olives
- Spinach
- Squash
- Sweet potato
- Turnips
- Yam
- Zucchini
- Kelp

OILS

- Olive oil
- Flax/hemp oil
- Grape seed oil
- Orange oil
- Coconut oil
- Sesame oil

GRAINS

- Amaranth
- Barley
- Buckwheat sprouts
- Wheat sprouts
- Kamut
- Millet
- Rye
- Oat groats
- Quinoa
- Ground flax
- Wheat (hard red)
- Wild Rice

Let's Get Started

SPICES & HERBS

Basil	Mexican chili pdr.
Cayenne	Mustard pdr.
Cinnamon	Nutmeg
Cloves	Onion pdr.
Coriander	Paprika
Cumin	Thyme
Dijon mustard	Pepper
Dill weed	Poultry ssng.
Fennel seeds	Sage
Garlic	Sun-dried olives
Italian ssng.	Curry paste
Kelp pdr.	

NUTS & SEEDS

Almonds	Pine nuts
Brazil nuts	Pistachio nuts
Cashews	Poppy seeds
Chia seeds	Psyllium seeds
Flax seeds	Sesame seeds
Ground flax	Sunflower seeds
Hazelnuts	Walnuts
Pecans	Soy nuts

FLAVOURINGS
Almond ext.
Pure vanilla ext.
Vanilla bean

LEGUMES
Adzuki
Lentils
Mung

NUT BUTTERS
Almond butter
Brazil nut butter
Cashew butter
Hazelnut butter
Sunflower butter

SEA PRODUCTS
Nori wraps
Wakami
Sea noodles
Sea vegetables
Sea vegetables

SPROUTING SEEDS
Alfalfa
Broccoli
Radishes

VINEGARS
White wine vin.
Red wine vin.
Apple cider vin.
Balsamic vin.

SWEETENERS

Agave	Dates
Yacon	Maple Syrup
Lakanto	Stevia
Coconut Sugar	Sucanat

In The Pantry!

Keep in mind that a large freezer is beneficial to store extra nuts, seeds, grains, tetra paks of coconut milk, and for fruits and vegetables, as well as for finished products such as nut burgers and herbed onion bread.

DRIED BEANS
Sprouting beans	Mung beans
Sprouting seeds	Peas - green or yellow
Adzuki beans	
Chickpeas	Pinto Beans
Lentils	
Lima beans	

DRIED FRUITS
Dates	Raisins
Figs	Cranberries
Prunes	Carob powder/nibs
Apricots	
Coconut	

RAW NUTS
Almonds	Pecan
Brazil Nuts	Pine nuts
Filberts	Walnuts
Macadamia nuts	

SEASONINGS
Sea salt	Apple cider vinegar
Peppercorn Dried	Braggs
Herbs	Balsamic
Spices	Nama shoyu
Tamari	

MISCELLANEOUS
Sauerkraut	Psyllium
Sea vegetables	Yeast flakes
Sea noodles	Supplements
Spices	Vitamins
Cocoa	Vanilla beans
Chia	etc.

SWEETENERS
Agave	Maple syrup
Nectar/syrup	Sucanat
Yacan syrup	Stevia

RAW SEEDS
Flax	Sesame
Pumpkin	Sunflower

WHOLE GRAINS
Raw oat groats	Quinoa
Raw buckwheat Groats	Wild rice

OILS
Coconut	Sesame
Flax	Sunflower
Olive oil	

CANNED GOODS
Organic tomatoes
Coconut milk
Organic beans

Shelf Life & Dry Storage of Seeds, Beans & Grains

SEED/BEAN/GRAIN	SHELF LIFE
Adzuki beans	5 years
Alfalfa seeds	4 Years
Almonds	4 Years
Arugula seeds	5 years
Barley (whole for grass)	2 Years
Barley, hulled	2 Years
Basil seeds	3 Years
Black turtle beans	5 years
Broccoli seeds	5 Years
Buckwheat, in hull	2 Years
Buckwheat, hulled (groats)	2 Years
Cabbage seeds	5 years
Cauliflower seeds	5 years
Celery seeds	5 years
Clover seeds, crimson	4 Years
Cress seeds, curly	5 years
Dill seeds	3 Years
Fennel (leaf)	3 Years
Fenugreek seeds	5 years
Flax seeds, brown	3 Years
Flax seeds, golden	3 Years
Garbanzo beans	5 years
Garlic chives	12-24 Months
Hemp Seeds	5 years
Kale seeds, Red Russian	5 years
Kamut kernels	2 Years
Leek*	12-24 Months
Lentils	5 years
Millet	5 years
Mizuna beans	5 years
Mung Beans	5 years
Oats, in hull	2 Years
Oats, hulled	2 Years
Onions	12-24 Months
Peas	5 years
Peanuts	5 years
Pinto beans	5 years
Popcorn	8 years

SEED/BEAN/GRAIN	SHELF LIFE
Pumpkin seeds	2 Years
Quinoa	3 Years
Radish seeds	5 years
Rice	3 Years
Rye kernels	2 Years
Sesame seeds	2 Years
Soy beans	4 Years
Spelt seeds	2 Years
Sunflower seeds, in shell	2 Years
Sunflower seeds, hulled	2 Years
Tatsoi seeds	5 years
Triticale seeds	2 Years
Wheat kernels, Hard Red Winter	2 Years

Soaking time for Nuts & Seeds

Enzyme inhibitors, phytates (phytic acid), polyphenols (tannins), and goitrogens prevent the nut from sprouting prematurely. Enzyme inhibitors come in two forms: digestive enzymes and metabolic enzymes. Digestive enzymes in our GI tract begin the process of breaking down the food. Metabolic enzymes help every biological process the body does. Enzyme inhibitors found on every grain, seed, nut and bean have the ability to clog the GI tract when consumed in large amounts. This enzyme inhibitor, "phytate," which is a phytic acid, reaps havoc on our GI tract, creating discomfort during digestion. When the enzyme inhibitor phytate has not been soaked before consumption, the untreated phytate can combine with calcium, magnesium, copper, iron and especially zinc in the intestinal tract and block their absorption. This leads to serious mineral deficiencies and bone loss, especially on the raw live vegan diet as these foods serve as a large portion of our intake. It would not be so noticeable in a mainstream diet, as the person would get minerals from animal based foods. To prevent deficiency, we soak our nuts in a solution of 1 tbsp of salt per 1L of water. This process activates the enzymes that then deactivate the enzyme inhibitors, allowing us to digest the nuts properly. Benefits of soaking nuts, seeds, grains and beans are plentiful. Soaking removes or reduces phytic acid and tannins. Soaking neutralizes the enzyme inhibitors, and encourages the production of beneficial enzymes. Soaking increases the amounts of vitamins, especially B vitamins and proteins due to breaking down of the protective coating. Soaking breaks down gluten making digestion easier. Soaking helps prevent mineral deficiencies and bone loss and helps neutralize toxins in the colon and keeps the colon clean. In layman's terms, think of Soaking as aiding digestion, like juicing, like chewing for long periods of time before swallowing, allowing the goodness of the food to be ready for absorption instead of just passing through with minimal benefit and maximum risk!

Soaking Nuts & Seeds

Nuts	Method	Soak Time	Rinse	Suggested Use
Almonds Brazil nuts Hazelnuts Pecans Walnuts	Use a 1l jar, top with warm filtered water add 1 tbsp of sea salt.	8-12 hours on counter.	Change the water once a day, do not add more sea salt. Nuts will keep in the fridge for 5 days, with water changed daily. Or, rinse and dehydrate at 118 degrees F. for 24 hours and store in air-tight container in refrigerator (no H2O).	Beverages, breads, nut cheeses, pates, crackers, desserts, dressings, entrees, salads, snacks, sauces.
Cashews	Use a 1l jar, top with warm filtered water add 1 tbsp of sea salt.	2-4 hours. The soak time for this nut is less than for any other, because it tends to get slimy Also, they have little life in them due to their harvesting method.	Drain and rinse, then dehydrate at 200-250 F until completely dry - about 24 hours. Remember, drying temp. isn't critical here due to the few enzymes in this nut.	Desert fillings Ice cream milk cream sauces
Sunflower Seeds	Use a 1l jar, top with warm filtered	15 mins - 1 hour is long enough for these.	Drain and rinse, and enjoy or feel free to dehydrate no higher than 118 degrees	Used in our Mock Chicken, Mock Tuna, and Olive Tapenade

Sprouting

Start with 3 large, wide-mouthed glass jars, a plastic mesh screen, some rubber bands, and a dish rack to sprout seeds. A colander/pot combination with a lid can be used for large beans, as they do best in a dark place. So, even though we are not cooking, we still have use for our pots. The trick here is sterile containers and clean water. If you're on town water with chlorine, opt for distilled water or get a filter for your tap to reduce or eliminate the chlorine.

Use a large stockpot with the strainer in it for sprouting your mung and adzuki beans. Put enough beans in the pot to just cover the bottom. Add enough water to cover the beans by an inch, and then set it on the counter. The next day pour the swollen beans from the pot into the strainer, and rinse them with fresh water. Pour the old water onto any houseplants that need watering. Clean the pot, place the rinsed beans that are still in the colander back into the pot, place a salad plate for weight onto the beans, and put the lid on the pot to make it dark. The strainer makes rinsing super easy, as you can lift the beans out of the water with the strainer and rinse them after the initial day of soaking. After day one, rinse 2 or 3 times daily, depending on the humidity in the house. If it is really dry, then rinse 3 times.

Use jars for seeds and small beans. Put 1 cup of sprouting beans or seeds into the jars and cover them well with water. Label each jar, and place them out of direct sunlight for the time specified on the sprouting chart. Then rinse every 8 hours and place them (still in the jar) on a dish rack, out of direct sunlight, on a 45-degree angle. This will allow the beans or seeds to stay moist and continue sprouting.

Sprouts are ready to eat when they sprout a stem that is twice the length of the bean itself, which is about one half to one inch in length. One inch is optimal. After the beans or seeds have fully sprouted, give them one final rinse, remove the hulls, and place the hulled sprouts into a colander to drain. Allow the cleaned sprouts to drain thoroughly before putting them in a glass container to be stored in the refrigerator. Don't close the lid on them, and be sure to rinse and drain the sprouts every couple of days. This will increase their expiration date from a few days to a week. Sprouts also store nicely in the green veggie bags that are designed to keep veggies fresh. They are at their optimum in nutrients during the first few days after sprouting.

You will soon get a handle on how many sprouts each person in your household consumes on a daily basis. I find that it takes four days to sprout, and that my husband and I consume all of it within that time frame. Use them in the Breakfast Green Shake, put them in hummus, add them to salad, use them at dinner, whether it is for a topping on a pizza, or as an addition to a soup, or part of the ingredients in Nori Wraps!

Remember, sprouts are live enzymes and oxygen rich, and your body craves them. Be cautious to the fact that broccoli, alfalfa, and radish seeds, etc. are so tiny that they sprout tiny hairs, which could easily be mistaken for mould. Continue to rinse them and place a lid back on them to keep them dark. In a day or two sprouting begins bearing two tiny leaves. Finish sprouting in indirect sunlight for the next 24 hours, to "green" the sprouts more.

I came across a sprouter that I especially like for sprouting small seeds. It's called a "Biosta Sprouter", and it's made in Canada. This three-tiered, stacking, round plastic container drains on each level. It is small, it sits on the counter and is perfect for sprouting tiny seeds. Each tiered level has tiny-ridged grooves, allowing it to hold approximately 2 tablespoons of water, even after draining. Each tier has a drain that pours down onto the tray below it, and on down to the bottom collection tray. Make sure to alternate trays, so that one tray's drain is not on top of the drain below it. If water seems to be trapped in one of the chambers, lift up the whole unit and tap it on the counter. This should eliminate any air lock in the drain. Due to the grooves in the bottom of the trays, you must be vigilant in your cleaning and rinsing before starting your next batch. The unit must be sterile each time you use it. Use 1 tablespoon of bleach per pint of water for sterilizing, then rinse well, and turn the sprouter upside down to dry.

Most of the time, Phil and I have seeds and beans at various stages of sprouting. We only stop sprouting before we travel. I use all of my drained water from my sprouts to feed my houseplants. I even fed my Christmas tree last year, and noticed that it lost very few needles and retained its beautiful, dark green color from December 12th to January 6th!

Sprouting Table

Legumes/ Seeds	Method	Soak Time	Rinse	Growing Time	Suggested Use
Adzuki, Chickpeas/ Garbanzo beans, Green peas, Kidney beans, Lentils, Mung Beans, Pinto beans, Soy beans	Jar	8-12 hours	2-3 times per day	3-4 days	Salads, casseroles, patés, soups
Alfalfa seeds, Clover, Radish seeds, Mustard seeds, Quinoa, Watercress seeds	Jar	6-8 hours	2-3 times per day	4-6 days. Should be green on last day.	Garnishes, salads, sandwiches, wraps, nori rolls
Broccoli seeds, Cabbage seeds, Fenugreek seeds, Kale seeds	Jar	6-8 hours	2-3 times per day	3-5 days. Should be green on last day.	Juices, salads, soup
Barley, Buckwheat, groats, in hull Sunflower seeds, in hull, Winter wheat, berries	Sprout in Jar then plant in soil	8-12 hours	2-3 times per day	Jar: 2-3 days Soil: 5 days	Soups
Barley, Buckwheat, groats, hulled Oat groats, Millet	Jar	8-12 hours	2-3 times per day	1 day	Cereals, cookies, crackers, salads

Let's Get Started

Legumes/Seeds	Method	Soak Time	Rinse	Growing Time	Suggested Use
Chia seeds, Flax seeds	Mixing bowl	12 hours Equal parts seeds to water	Chia seeds, Flax seeds	N/A	12 hours Equal parts seeds to water
Onion seeds	Jar	4-6 hours	3 times per day	6-8 days. Should be green on last day.	Garnish, salad, breads, crackers, nori rolls, wraps
Corn kernels	Jar	20 hours	2-3 times per day	4-6 days. Should green on last day	Entree, salads, soup
Lettuce seeds	Jar		2-3 times per day	4-6 days. Should green on last day	Garnishes, salads, sandwiches
Oats	Jar	1 hour	1-2 times per day	3-4 days	Salads
Wild Rice	Jar	4 days wash before soaking.	2 times per day		Rice pilaf

"Raw Food 101"
Terminology & Sources

One store may not contain everything you need, but you can substitute. If you have 60-70% of the product listed in your recipe, considering the abundance of oils and sweeteners, it will turn out. Check out the section on Science Behind the Food for an in-depth look at recommended fruits and vegetables.

Agar: A natural jelling and thickening agent made from seaweed. Available in all health food stores and in some major whole food grocers.

Agave Nectar/Syrup: A sweetener extracted from the inner core of blue agave, a cactus- like plant. Agave is absorbed slowly into the blood stream so there are no highs or lows in blood sugar. As it is unprocessed, the vitamins and minerals in Agave nectar and syrup are still present. It can be found in many health food stores or in the health food section of major grocers.

Apple Cider Vinegar with Mother: This vinegar is an organic raw apple cider vinegar made from the finest organic apples, full of zesty natural goodness and contains the amazing "mother" of vinegar which occurs naturally as connected strand-like chains of protein enzyme molecules and is highly regarded throughout history. This product is not new, is as old as 400 B.C. Hippocrates, the Father of Medicine, used it for its amazing natural cleansing, healing and energizing health qualities. Use it on salads, veggies, etc. My puppies even get a tsp. once a day for their optimal health!! I recommend Braggs organic Raw Apple Cider Vinegar as one of the best out there!

Arrowroot powder: Used as a thickening agent. Available in health food stores.

Blue-Green Algae: See spirulina.

Butters: Almond, Brazil nut, Cashew, Hazelnut, Macadamia and sunflower. Thick, cold-pressed from organic raw nuts. Available in health food stores and in the health food section of major grocers.

Cacao Beans: Raw Cacao Beans or nibs. The nibs are taken from peeled and broken seeds (or beans) of the cacao fruit, from which all chocolate products are made. Buy in raw form only. This product is found in many health food stores or in the health food section of major grocers.

Cacao Butter: Pure cold pressed oil of the cacao bean. White chocolate is made with cacao butter. Found in most health food stores and in the health food section of major grocers.

Carob Powder: Made from a raw, brown, pod shaped fruit found in Mediterranean countries. It is used as a substitute for chocolate, and has no caffeine. Buy in raw form only. Carob powder may also be substituted in chocolate recipes. It is found in health food stores and in the health food section of major grocers.

Cacao Powder: Comes from cacao beans. Buy in organic form only. Cacao powder is used in chocolate recipes, and found in health food stores or in the health food section of major grocers.

Chia Seeds: A gluten free grain. Chia seeds come from the chia plant, which was used as a staple in the Mayan and Aztec civilizations. They have twice the amount of protein of many other grains, three times the antioxidants of blueberries, five times more calcium than milk, and three times more iron than spinach! Sprinkle chia seeds into a glass of cold water or ice tea, and drink it. But don't leave it in your drink for too long or they will gel. Chia is also a great soup thickener, and can be sprinkled on salads or soups. Available in all health food stores.

Chickpeas: Also known as garbanzo or ceci beans, used for sprouting or making hummus. It is available in the bean section of health food stores or at major grocers.

Coconuts: Readily available at whole food, health food and Asian markets.

Coconut butter/oil: Oil pressed from the flesh of coconuts, sometimes called coconut oil. Smell before using; it should smell like a fresh coconut. If it smells burnt, then it may have gone rancid. This will ruin your recipe. Available in health food stores and in the health food section of major grocers.

Coconut Sugar: 100% pure organic crystallized coconut sap from Thailand. It's harvested from the sap of unopened coconut blossoms; there are no additives, no bleaching and no stripping of minerals or nutrients. It's not raw due to boiling, but it's healthy; low glycemic index of 35, 12% sugar, high in potassium, magnesium, zinc and iron, and high in several key B vitamins.

Dried Fruits: Read packages to be sure that it is organic and dried without sulphur and sugar. Can be found in health food stores or in the health food section of major grocers. You can also dry your own in a dehydrator. Make sure to slice the fruit and place on a Teflon sheet. Do not dry fruit on racks.

Galangal: A good substitute is fresh ginger. Found in Asian Markets.

Goji Berries: The goji berry is a deep-red fruit that is picked and dried before consumption. A dried goji berry is as small as a raisin. It contains all eight essential amino acids and up to twenty-one trace minerals. It also contains the richest carotenoids on earth, and 500 times the vitamin C, by weight, of oranges. Vitamins include B1, B2, B6 and vitamin E. The Goji berry is regarded as the key to longevity!

Grains and Seeds: Make sure they have not been processed, or they will not sprout. They are available in most health food stores and in the health food section of major grocers. You can also buy online at www.westcoastseeds.com.

Greens Plus **Vitamineralgreen, Life's Greens:** A nutrient-dense super food containing a full spectrum of naturally occurring absorbable vitamins, minerals, and trace elements. *Greens Plus* also contains all of the essential amino acids, antioxidants, fatty acids, chlorophyll, soluble and insoluble fibers and other organic nutrients required for optimal health. They can be found in health food Stores and in the supplements and health food section of major grocers. A good online source is: www.puritanpride.com.

Made from raw organic hemp seeds: Hemp protein is a balanced whole protein, rich in essential fatty acids, amino acids, vitamins, minerals and antioxidants. It provides a perfect balance of Omega-3. The seeds contain 33% pure digestible protein and are rich in vitamin E, omega-3, and omega-6 essential fatty acids. Hemp is good! It is available in health food stores or in the health food section of major grocers.

Honey, raw: A natural sweetener, available in health food stores and in the health food section of major grocers.

Irish Moss: A seaweed currently harvested on the coast of Ireland, Canada's Maritime Provinces, and Jamaica. It is used as a thickener to bind desserts and cheeses. Soak 12-24 hours before using in recipes.

Kaffir Lime Leaves: Bright green leaves from the Kaffir Lime Tree found in Southeast Asia. They add a citrus tang and floral aroma to recipes. They can be grown in any climate, but must be wintered indoors. Found in large health food stores and in Asian markets.

Lakanto: An all-natural sweetener that looks and tastes like sugar, derived from the luohan guo fruit from China. The fruit combined with erythritol is specially fermented from non-GMO corn so that you can trust it. May people have trouble digesting foods with sugar alcohol but not the case with this one as it is fermented, so no gas, diarrhea or bloating all due to fermentation where other sugar alcohols are made from hydrogenation. Available in upscale health food stores and some major upscale grocers that house a health food section or on-line at kellyorganics.com

Lecithin: A powder found in many health food stores. Make sure it is not made from non-GMO soy.

Liquid Aminos: Braggs Liquid Aminos, similar in taste to soy sauce, not heated or pasteurized, used as a flavoring in place of salt. Available at The Bulk Barn, in health food stores and in the health food section of major grocers.

Maca: Known for its strength and stamina enhancer; also known to stabilize blood pressure, as it lowers high blood pressure and raises low blood pressure. Found in powder or capsule form. Available in health food stores and in the supplements and health food sections of major grocers.

Macadamia Nut Oil: You can make it yourself, if you have a really good "Angel Food Processor." You can buy it at an upscale health food store or on line at www.macnutoil.com. If this doesn't work, substitute for another nut oil.

Mesquite Powder: From the mesquite tree. The seedpods are gathered and ground into a fine powder. It has a molasses like flavor, with a hint of caramel. It is high in protein; calcium; magnesium; potassium; iron; and zinc. Available in health food stores and in the health food section of major grocers.

Manna Bread: Found in the freezer food isle of your major grocer or in health food stores with a freezer section. Great if you are out of time to make your own.

Maple Sugar Powder: Dehydrated maple syrup; a natural sweetener. Available in health food stores and in the health food section of major grocers.

Microgreens: *Greens Plus* - Greens contain all of the essential amino acids, antioxidants, fatty acids, chlorophyll, soluble and insoluble fibers and other organic nutrients required for optimal health. Many green powders are available in health food stores and in the health food section of major grocers. Buy online at: www.puritanpride.com.

Miso: A thick paste made from soybeans, grain and sea salt. Used as a flavoring. Miso is unpasteurized and naturally aged, and contains enzymes. It is available in dark, light, and medium, in jars or packets. Available in health food stores and in the health food section of major grocers.

Nama Shoyu: An organic unpasteurized soy sauce, aged in wooden kegs from the wheat grain. If you want a non-wheat product, use Braggs. Nama Shoyu is bottled and can be found in upscale health foods.

Nutritional Yeast: Found in powder form. If you have Celiac disease make sure the source of your nutritional yeast is derived from beet. Available at The Bulk Barn, in health food stores and in the health food section of major grocers.

Nuts, Raw Organic: Almonds, Cashews, Filberts, Macadamia, Pecans, Pistachio, Sesame, Soy, and Walnuts. Make sure they are raw and organic. Available at The Bulk Barn, in bulk at health food stores, or packaged in the health food section of major grocers.

Oat groats, raw: Be sure to buy un-steamed oats for cereal, flour and raw food recipes. Available in health food stores and in the health food section of major grocers.

Oils: Flaxseed, Hemp, Olive, Nut & Seed oils are available in most whole food grocers and in specialty health food stores.

Olives, raw organic: Available in most health food stores or in the health food section of major grocers.

Psyllium: The husks of psyllium seeds are ground to a powder and are used as a thickener. Buy only a very finely ground powder.

Pure water: Any filtered, distilled, reverse osmosis or artesian spring water.

Sea Salt: Harvested by hand. Mineral-rich, not chemically processed. Sun and wind dried, which locks in the ocean's vital trace elements. Readily available in the spice aisle or in the health food section at most grocers, and definitely in all health food stores.

Sea Vegetables: Dulse, reddish in color, dried. Kelp, in noodle form. Nori, a sea algae flattened into black sheets, used in sushi. Wakame, dried and in black spice form, found in Miso soup and packaged dry. Can be used in salad. Arama is another sea vegetable. It is a brown, lacey algae. Introduce sea vegetables to ensure iodine uptake. Available in some major health food stores, or online at: www.seatanglenoodle.com.

Spices: Use fresh organic whenever you can. Dried and packaged is good, readily available and marked organic. Available in all health food and in most whole food stores.

Spirulina: A fine powder dried from blue- green algae, rich in vitamins, minerals and phytonutrients. This micro algae is 60% all vegetable protein, rich in beta-carotene, iron, and vitamin B12, the vitamin we tend to be lax in on the raw live vegan plan. I supplement my *Greens Plus* shake with a tablespoon of spirulina. I also use liquid B12 and place a tincture under my tongue. Available in all health food stores or online at: www.puritanpride.com.

Stevia: A sweetener made from the stevia flower. Far sweeter than sugar. Found in powdered or liquid form. Stevia is the best alkaline sweetener on the market today. Available in health food stores and in the health food section of major grocers.

Sucanat: Dehydrated, unprocessed sugar cane. Available in juice or crystal form. Found in all health food stores and at major grocers.

Tahini: A smooth, thick butter made from hulled sesame seeds. High in calcium and protein. Available in Asian markets, in most health food stores and in the health food section of major grocers.

Tamari: A wheat free soy sauce, unpasteurized, no alcohol added. Available in all health food Stores, at major grocers and in Asian markets.

Tempeh: A cultured food made from soybeans and sometimes grains. Read labels for source ingredients. Available in all health food stores and in Asian markets.

Ume Vinegar: A ruby red, tangy, salty vinegar, made from pickling umeboshi plums with sea salt and shiso leaves. Available whole, in paste or vinegar form, in most upscale health food stores.

Vanilla Beans/Extract: The actual pod is best. Slit the pod and remove the tiny beans. A little goes a long way flavor wise. I cut off an inch at a time. The left over pod can be used in vodka or bourbon or light rum or brandy to make your own vanilla extract! Available in all health food stores and in the baking section of whole food grocers.

Vinegars: Apple cider made from aged apple cider, rich in enzymes and potassium. Apple cider vinegar should be raw, organic and unpasteurized. Available in most health foods stores and in the health food section of major grocers.

Wasabi: This hot, tangy Japanese horseradish paste comes in a tube, jar or loose powder. Available in health food stores, at major grocers and in Asian markets.

Yacon Syrup: A sweetener derived from the roots of the yacon plant, yacon syrup is a good source of antioxidants. Contains Fructo-oligosaccharide, or FOS, which the body cannot process, so it passes through without leaving behind absorbable sugar compounds. Yacon is glucose free and often recommended for diabetics or those at risk of becoming diabetic. Available in few upscale health food stores or online at: www.sunFood.com and www.navitasnaturals.com.

Foods to Avoid

Beverages: Calorie-laden beverages such as alcoholic drinks, fancy coffees, milkshakes and soda pop.

Deep-fried foods: French fries, fried chicken, fried fish, onion rings, anything fried.

Fatty meats: hamburger, pork chops, spare ribs, cold cuts, processed meats, canned meats, luncheon meats, hotdogs.

High-fat dairy products: cheese, cream, cream cheese, ice cream, sour cream, whipping cream, whole milk, butter.

High-salt convenience foods: canned and pre-packaged soups and stews, macaroni and cheese in a box, ramen noodles, anything with MSG: salty fried snack foods, cheese puffs, corn chips, potato chips.

Pre-packaged processed foods with infinite shelf life containing hydrogenated fat or lard and refined starch and sugars: cookies pastries, crackers margarine, pastries, pies, microwave popcorn, breads corn syrup, white sugar and other sugars such as glucose, high fructose, white flour, white rice and other refined starches.

Our goal is to consume at least 80% Raw Food. So if there is something in the "Foods to Avoid" section you would like to have, then perhaps you will re-think how to incorporate it into that 20%. Some of us will adopt the raw live vegan lifestyle at a higher level; this is fine too. Some embrace the program 100%. I personally am higher than 80%, but then again that is a personal choice.

On my journey towards wellness, the more I read, the more I realize chemically laden processed foods must become a thing of the past. A healthy GI tract requires proper food choices. I thought that buying healthy low fat snacks from the health food section of my grocery store was as good as it gets. I never thought twice about the chemical preservatives, artificial sweeteners and MSG they contain. I now know differently. Foods on the Raw Live Vegan program have a definite shelf life and a short one at that. You will come to appreciate foods that actually begin to decay in days, knowing that they are natural and that your body will not have to work so hard to digest them. There is no waste on this program. When vegetables start to break down, simply juice them. When bananas get too dark, peel and freeze them; they make a great base for ice cream or your breakfast smoothie.

Why not dairy?

One percent of our calcium travels through our blood. Those who drink the most dairy have the poorest bone density, due to the fact that dairy is high in sulphur, which causes the blood to become too acidic. Dairy has been attributed to a surprising number of health problems including diarrhea, constipation, blood sugar imbalance, eczema, acne, digestive problems, chronic sinus and ear infections, and PMS. Milk is also linked to teenage acne and colic in babies. Milk fat has been identified as a cholesterol elevating fat because it contains cholesterol that is primarily saturated.

Calcium is important to our health for blood clotting, nerve function, muscle contraction, and to regulate heart rhythm.

All the nutrients dairy offers can be found in plant life without the fat. The disease fighting nutrients found in plant food and not available in milk products is an added bonus. The depletion of our stores of calcium in our bones and the inability to get the required amount of calcium from cooked foods leaves us open to arthritis. Good calcium levels are measured by how little you use (as evidenced in bone density through testing) and not by how much dairy you consume. I can remember being diagnosed lactose intolerant at the age of 40 and feeling a sense of impending doom, as I thought dairy was such an important component of my diet. My Internist laughed and assured me I would get adequate calcium with a calcium supplement taken with vitamin D, which aids calcium absorption. He also recommended increasing my intake of dark leafy vegetables that contain calcium and are lower in fat, sugar and calories. Dark green vegetables contain other important vitamins such as vitamin C, which aids the immune system, acts as an antioxidant and an anti-inflammatory. Folate is also present in dark green leafy vegetables. It is necessary for the formation of red blood cells and reduces the risk of heart disease and some cancers. I all but laughed when reading raw food diet books and their recommendation to give up dairy. They took me back to that day when my internist said, "Trust Me! You are better off without it!"

Why not meat?

All proteins, cooked or raw, require an acidic environment for proper digestion. This is where raw food is superior to cooked food. The cooking process alters protein molecules and makes them difficult to digest. Heat in excess of 118 degrees Fahrenheit destroys active enzymes. Grilling, broiling and frying is devastating to your health as these cooking methods create advanced glycosylation end products, which

Let's Get Started

trigger inflammation, such as arthritis and other inflammatory diseases.

Animal proteins and inorganic dairy products have high levels of toxic chemicals and artificial hormones introduced directly by the farmer to stimulate growth. This has lead to many major diseases afflicting unsuspecting consumers of these products. How many meat recalls have you witnessed lately? Chlorophyll is a safe, natural source of protein present in plant life. It gives plants their green or purple colour, and is only available in its natural state in live food. Chlorophyll has been used to treat ulcers, skin disease and bad breath. Pharmaceutical companies have tried to bottle it, to treat these and other conditions, but have found that it becomes unstable. As chlorophyll cannot be reproduced synthetically, pharmacists continue to use antibiotics to treat these same conditions. Proteins derived from raw food sources require less energy and enzyme activity to break down the loosened peptide bonds that hold the amino acids in place. This makes it easier for the body to digest and absorb it.

In an unmonitored high protein diet, note the key word *unmonitored*. There are cases where certain people afflicted with certain disorders actually benefit from a high protein animal-based diet, where their physician closely monitors their diet, designing to meet their specific nutritious needs. However, for the everyday person consuming an exorbitant amount of animal-based protein, this type of diet may cause kidney damage, gout, and increased cholesterol and triglyceride levels stressing the major organs, including the heart and liver. As animal protein is low in fibre, it will sit in the digestive tract, leading to constipation, due to the meat source coming from animals fed a low-grain diet. If you must eat meat, buy from a certified organic-grain fed supplier and keep your consumption to less than 20% of your weekly diet.

Also, poaching and stewing are preferable to grilling, broiling and frying. Fish is preferable to meat, as it has about 25% less advanced glycosylation end products than steak or chicken. Research has shown that diabetics who ate a diet high in advanced glycosylation end products (AGEs) had a 35% jump in inflammation related diseases. (Note the acronym for advanced glycosylation end products spells out AGE!) Nothing will age you faster than cooking at high heat. Let's not forget that consumption of animal proteins throws our body into an acidic state forcing it to neutralize this food by pulling minerals from our organs and bones.

The best proteins are derived from green leafy vegetables, sprouted nuts, grains, seeds, and legumes (beans) – all of which are higher alkaline-forming foods. Wheatgrass juice is not only a wonderful source of protein, but is also known for its detoxifying benefits to the body and its powerful cleansing properties. We buy organic from a reputable source and sprout our own protein. This way we control the source of our water and sprout in sterile conditions.

Why not sugar?

Refined sugars are simple carbohydrates that provide calories but are low in vitamins, minerals and fibre. Refined sugar puts great stress on the pancreas, which at best struggles to balance the sugar levels with insulin. Sugar destroys B vitamins, creates problems with digestion and enlarges the liver, as witnessed with alcohol consumption. Sugar promotes Candida, a yeast infection. Sugar reaps havoc on metabolism by affecting the thyroid gland. It weakens the immune system thereby leaving us susceptible to cancer. White sugar, brown sugar, molasses, and processed honey are in the low to medium acid range, tipping the pH balance to more acidic if you consume too much of these products. This will inevitably leave you prone to osteoporosis, due to bone loss because the body borrows calcium from the bones in order to balance pH. Sugar is very addictive. It was considered a drug in Victorian times.

Why not sugar substitutes?

NutraSweet, Equal, Aspartame, Sweet 'N Low: these artificial sweeteners are at the high end of the acidic range, much higher than even refined sugar. This leaves the body prone to being in a state of chronic acidosis. With the alternative (so-called) *healthy choices* we assumed we made for ourselves and our families, we zeroed-in on their low caloric content; artificial sweeteners are truly a lame attempt of food scientists to remove sugar. But rest assured the products are high in fat! We also have fat-free products on the market that are high in sugar! The sugar substitute Aspartame, found in NutraSweet and Equal, is an unnatural substance produced by large chemical manufacturers. Aspartame is a neurotoxin that destroys brain cells. The body breaks it down into formaldehyde, which is a known cancer-causing agent. Aspartame has been linked to brain tumors, mood disorders, declining mental function, migraine headaches, and the list goes on! Splenda (sucralose) is no better. Splenda is an unnatural chemical substance synthesized by adding chlorine molecules to sugar. Chlorinated hydrocarbons found in the petrochemical industry are known carcinogens. Sucralose is a chlorinated hydrocarbon! Buzzwords abound in the food world, words like *Lite, Sugar-Free, Fat- Free* and the like – it's a wonder we are not all deaf!

Why not refined carbohydrates?

Refined carbohydrates – such as bread and pasta derived from white flour or refined white rice – are unhealthy, as they are acid forming. Also, the digestive system breaks down refined carbohydrates into sugar. Through this process our pancreas releases a rush of insulin to move the sugar from our bloodstream into our cells. Carbohydrates also boost serotonin – the feel good hormone – thus inducing a *high* from the spike in blood sugar, followed by a crash. Over time, this perpetuates hormonal imbalances. When we consume too many simple carbohydrates, our body stores the excess as fat. This happens even when we consume mainly fat free products. When we consume this type of carbohydrate and get the blood sugar spike and drop, we experience headaches, nausea, fatigue, mental confusion and hunger. Then we get hungry again and eat what we crave: more carbohydrates. And the vicious cycle of eating and craving begins. The continual stress on our pancreas and adrenal glands keeps our insulin levels chronically elevated. This promotes weight gain and increases our risk of diabetes, heart disease and more. Amazingly, when we are off these carbohydrates the craving stops.

Why not alcohol?

Because your body recognizes alcohol as sugar, the same rationale applies as to why not to consume sugar. Alcohol is an acid-forming beverage. It has been known to increase the risk of breast cancer in women as it increases estrogen levels. This results in as few as 3 glasses of wine a week. The consumption of alcohol while on estrogen therapy, such as oral estradiol, increases the risk of breast cancer because this combination doubles the amount of estrogen in the bloodstream. Studies for men showed increased estrogen levels with regular consumption of alcohol, which speaks volumes for their lack of libido. Enjoy the occasional drink, but not on a daily basis; there is still a 20% food choice to pull from the list if an 80% raw live vegan lifestyle is implemented. Save wine for special occasions. Hopefully they are not more than once a week, and know that if they are, they will have a negative impact on estrogen levels and libido. Recent studies show that red wine has beneficial effects on the heart by helping to keep arteries clear. The supplement industry has put the red wine supplement called *Reservatrol* in capsule form.

Why not Hydrogenated, Saturated, or trans-fatty Fats?

Saturated fats cannot be broken down by our digestive system efficiently. Saturated, hydrogenated fats are believed to clog veins and arteries. This creates sluggishness in the lymphatic system, which slows the removal of toxins. It also slows down the circulatory and respiratory systems. As these two systems work in tandem to pump oxygen into our bloodstream, the overall effect makes our heart work harder, leaves us feeling short of breath, tired and lethargic. Saturated fats, the bad fats, raise LDL (bad cholesterol) leading to high blood pressure and heart disease.

We need fats to be healthy, but we need the right types of fats. Saturated, hydrogenated and trans-fats are not it.

Why not caffeine?

When we drink caffeine we increase our adrenaline, which breaks down lean body tissue. The less lean body tissue we have the lower our metabolism. Increased adrenaline blocks estrogen receptors and increases insulin levels. Since insulin is the fat-storing hormone, we don't want to drink caffeine with a meal because it will store the extra fat in the fat reserves, which we work so hard to deplete. Caffeine initially increases serotonin. It then creates the crash, which makes us crave carbohydrates. Coffee has been linked as a benefit health-wise in studies that have shown reduction in prostate cancer, Parkinson's disease, diabetes, cirrhosis of liver, gallstones, kidney stones and Alzheimer's. When my son was small and suffered childhood asthma the doctor recommended a few sips of black coffee as coffee is related to theophylline, an old asthma medication used to improve asthma symptoms. Coffee and black teas are acid-forming beverages; so if you must have that second cup, neutralize it with a stevia sweetener. There will always be controversy over certain foods and beverages, and too much of anything equates to disaster. Again, knowing you have freedom to choose 20% of your food consumption from the "Foods to Avoid" list, caffeine may be the one to kick-off your day!

Cravings

Many of the foods we crave – whether it's chocolate, coffee, carbohydrates, sugar or fast foods – all have one thing in common: they all contain addictive substances. This makes them as addictive as alcohol or drugs. The food industry, with its use of such additives as sugar, corn syrup, salt and MSG, has made food highly addictive. Fast food restaurants and companies that produce pre-packaged convenience foods profit at the expense of our expanding waistlines! Physical cravings are a response to hunger. When we eat a poor diet, based on convenience foods, we create internal imbalance and damage the micro-flora of our GI tract, leaving us prone to bacteria and yeast infections.

Allergens, when consumed, cause cravings, as the body craves what it should not put into it. This works like an addiction. One of the leading allergens in food is contained in dairy products. Other allergens are contained in eggs, fish, shellfish, peanuts, tree nuts and soy.

Fermented foods such as sauerkraut and vinegars, even apple cider vinegar, are good for restoring health to the GI tract.

Probiotics, such as Lactobacillus and Acidophilus, are often recommended to treat Candida and to restore health to the GI tract. Studies show that supplementing probiotics protects the body against colon cancer.

If we are going to heal ourselves from the inside out, then it is important to get a thorough physical checkup to ensure success as we adopt a healthier way of eating. There is nothing more defeating than adopting a healthy lifestyle that may actually work against us due to an underlying health issue. Something as simple as a food allergy can prevent a person from achieving optimal health.

Emotional cravings occur through mental associations with food. Typically they are a response to stressors or triggers. When we are stressed, we resort to certain comfort foods, such as ice cream or donuts. If we have had a bad day at work, we might go for that glass of wine and then nachos and cheese. The aroma of a nearby bakery may give rise to a craving for freshly baked bread, even though we're not hungry. Seeing a plate of cookies on the kitchen counter might remind us that we really must have one.

It's important to face your emotions and allow yourself to feel them, as opposed to smothering them with food. If you're sad, allow yourself to cry. If you're frustrated, allow yourself time for a nice cup of green tea. Or sit down with pen and paper and list strategies to alleviate this frustration. Once you have listed some steps, you will feel empowered by your new inner strength. You will have dealt with your emotions in a constructive manner. This is so much better than filling your face with food and hating yourself for it later. And we all know that feeling! Also, allow yourself to bring joy into your life by knowing what you desire and opening yourself up to receiving it. This may mean obtaining new knowledge, starting a hobby or adopting a pet.

Sometimes we associate certain foods with celebrations. This is where physical and emotional needs collide, making the cravings more difficult to resist. Traditional holidays that we enjoy with family and friends are often celebrated with excessive food. This association of traditional food with a certain holiday makes it difficult to replace traditional family recipes with healthy choices. We risk upsetting those near to us if we break with tradition. Christmas would not be Christmas without chocolates, candy, fruitcake, trifle or rum cake. Hanukkah would not be Hanukkah without potato latkes, yeast donuts and Hanukkah cookies.

By adopting the raw live vegan lifestyle and preparing meals that nourish our bodies, the foods we leave behind are some of the most acidic on the pH chart, such as sugar, coffee, aspartame, milk, processed foods and meats. Eating a balanced, nutritious diet that is more alkaline and less acidic helps us to reduce cravings. When we incorporate the 80% rule in the raw live vegan lifestyle, we pair a glass of wine with fruit, vegetables and hummus. And if we simply have to have a cheese, goat's cheese would be the best choice. Also, feta is available in a number of textures ready to serve. Once you achieve a properly nourished body, on a consistent basis, you will no longer experience cravings!

With defining cravings, let's look at how we can deal with them as we work towards optimal health. Proper hydration with water and/or herbal teas helps prevent cravings. When we are dehydrated, our mind confuses thirst for hunger. As foods contain fluids and as our body does not care where it gets its' hydration, it may send out a signal for food when really we are thirsty. So be sure to drink water and if you feel hungry, try a warm cup of herbal tea and wait a few minutes to see if the craving passes.

Time is an important factor in cravings. Set your timer or peer at your watch and give yourself twenty minutes the next time you experience a craving. While you wait, grab your journal and write down what it feels like at that moment, then review your intake for the day. If you are on target for your daily food intake, then review your goals. Ask yourself if you're eating enough. Consider whether you are in such a hurry to get to a goal that you are skimping at your regular mealtime. If you are not getting enough food, you are not nourishing your body for optimal health. Also, a diet restricted in calories will cause your metabolism to slow down as your body preserves energy. So skimping on meals is really counterproductive to losing weight and gaining health.

Sleep is an important factor in overall health. Sleep patterns affect metabolism and energy and can also influence cravings. If you are overtired from lack of sleep your body becomes stressed; and stress induces cravings particularly for high calorie carbohydrates. Sometimes we have difficulty dealing with the new surge of energy that comes with eating the foods on this program. At the end of the day we still feel vibrant and find it hard to settle down. A supplement melatonin is a great natural aid I use when I travel and change time zones. It is safe compared to its chemical counterpart and quickly puts me back on track.

Hobbies are always nice too: enjoyable pastimes that can distract you from thoughts of food. Make sure you are not so distracted that your hobby overtakes your mealtime and leaves you hungry. This is when cravings can really kick in. But if you do miss a meal, perhaps hummus with flax crackers and veggies could hold you over until the next one.

The whole thing about adopting a new food program is knowing your likes and dislikes, trying to substitute allowable ingredients and creating dishes with your favorite tastes and textures. Being prepared with a variety of healthy foods and ingredients to work with will help prevent making wrong choices.

I read an amazing article written by Dr. Colleen Huber on "Cravings" on www.naturopathyworks.com. Her article (which she granted me permission to share in this book), suggests that when we crave certain foods our diet may be depleted of a certain mineral. If we include the depleted mineral in our diet, we will be successful in eliminating these cravings. Check out the following cravings and see if they apply to you. Then try to include the recommended mineral in your diet and see if it makes a difference. I pay the utmost attention to blood work, the tell-all of depleted nutrients and minerals. Then I refer to the charts found under our Vitamins, Minerals and Supplement section to see how I can add more into my diet to correct the depletion. Note in the following craving categories the emphasis is on *may* when it comes to a possible lacking of a particular food item in your diet. The final analysis is the definitive blood work. Sometimes our cravings are impulse or habit, but I found this article of interest and found it most worthy of sharing; sure beats setting a timer for twenty minutes to figure out if the craved food is for real or just an impulse!

If you crave coffee or tea your body may be lacking phosphorous, sulfur, salt or iron. In this case, try herbal teas accompanied with a real source of the deficient mineral such as nuts, beans, cruciferous vegetables, sea salt, apple cider vinegar, black cherries, seaweed and greens.

If you crave chocolate your body may be lacking magnesium. Good sources of magnesium are raw nuts, seeds, legumes, red beets, and fruits.

If you crave sweets your body may be lacking chromium, carbon, phosphorous, sulfur or tryptophan. Chromium is found in broccoli, grapes and dried beans. Carbon is found in fresh fruits. Phosphorus is found in nuts, legumes and grains. Sulfur is contained in cranberries, horseradish, cruciferous vegetables such as kale and cabbage. Tryptophan can be found in raisins, sweet potato and spinach.

If you crave bread and toast your body may be lacking nitrogen, found in nuts and beans.

If you crave oily snacks and fatty foods your body may be lacking calcium, found in mustard and turnip greens, broccoli, kale, legumes and sesame seeds.

If you crave alcohol and recreational drugs, your body may be lacking protein, avenin, calcium, glutamine or potassium. Protein is found in nuts. Avenin is contained in granola and oatmeal. Calcium is found in mustard turnip greens, broccoli, kale, legumes and sesame seeds. Glutamine can be sourced in a supplement such as glutamine powder or raw cabbage juice. Potassium can be found in sun-dried black olives, seaweed or bitter greens.

If you crave ice, your body may be lacking iron, found in seaweed, greens and black cherries.

If you crave burned foods, your body may be lacking carbon, found in fresh fruits.

Bad Cow

Both of my children were breastfed. I prepared their food fresh daily by pureeing fruits and vegetables. As breast milk is the most alkaline food on the pH chart, both kids blossomed and had great health, until they were introduced to dairy milk. Dairy is the most acidic food on the pH chart.

My daughter, Anna-Liesa, was introduced to dairy when she was eight months old. By the time she was three, she had developed asthma and Irritable Bowel Syndrome (IBS). At first, our doctor attributed these conditions to food sensitivities. He said that she would know which foods made her ill, and recommended that she avoid them. We already knew that she was allergic to soy. This ruled-out such prepared foods as bread products, cereals, margarine, and candy as they contain soy lecithin. Anna-Liesa naturally avoided foods that were high in fat, as they caused discomfort. These included theatre popcorn, and dairy products such as butter, ice cream, and cream-based desserts. Our daughter had a love-hate relationship with food. The rich, aromas tempted her, but the foods themselves caused severe abdominal cramps and discomfort that left her wondering which ingredient was the culprit. Ultimately, it was the dairy!

Our son Bryan's health problems started much earlier than our daughter's. At birth, he weighed 9 lbs 11 3/4 oz. Bryan, a real bruiser and one hungry little guy, like his sister, was breastfed. At four months I introduced pabulum to Bryan. But he was still so hungry all the time that he wouldn't give up his midnight feeding until he reached 5 months of age. This is when I started to supplement his feeding with cow's milk. I gave him one or two feedings with breast milk each day, and then I gave him a bottle. Subsequent to this, I slowly introduced him to fruits and vegetables. Over this same period, I weaned him off of breast milk, so that by six months of age, Bryan was drinking only cow's milk in addition to his pablum and other pureed foods. This allowed me to sleep at night and Bryan to thrive, which benefitted both of us, or so I thought. At his nine-month medical check-up, our doctor discovered that Bryan's liver was twice its normal size. By this time he had been off breast milk and onto cow's milk for three months. He was also refusing his meals. Our doctor was sure that this was because Bryan drank so much milk that it filled him up. He recommended that I take him completely off of cow's milk, and offer him only water, in a *sippy-cup*, with his baby food. He assured me that Bryan would miss one meal, at most, as he held out for his milk, and that I should stick with the plan, as Bryan would eventually eat. He was right; Bryan did not starve. He fussed a little over missing his dairy milk, and then he readily accepted the baby food that I had prepared for him. The result of all of this was that his liver returned to normal size.

One week later, I reintroduced Bryan to milk, in proper proportion to his solid food, and never gave it another thought. That is, until seventeen years later, when I found myself in the hospital at my son's bedside, watching him fight for his life, for thirty days. Parvovirus had attacked his liver and threatened to shut it down.

At the time my mind was on the present; I didn't think back to Bryan's earlier episode. Thinking back now, it seemed Bryan's liver had functioned just close enough to 'normal' over the span of seventeen years that nothing had been picked up. And as he appeared to thrive, like any other growing boy, no one expressed any concerns. Over that same period, his liver had been burdened with the task of processing dairy products, which weakened it. And as viruses always attack the weakest organ, the parvovirus attacked his liver. Animals can be inoculated against parvovirus, but not humans. Bryan's liver was failing so precipitously, and his condition had become so critical, he was placed at the top of the liver transplant list. On the Friday of his third week there, a match was found. If he survived the weekend, his doctors assured me, he would be prepped for surgery that Monday.

Bryan was a popular, outgoing 17-year old, well known in our tiny community. A great rally of support took place, and every church congregation and high school student and staff member congregated at the United Church, in Windsor, Nova Scotia, where we lived, and prayed for his recovery. Phil and I joined in too. We prayed for a miracle, as Bryan's condition was so tenuous that we thought we were going to lose him. And, for the first time in my life, I made a pact with God. I promised him that if he would give me back my Bryan, and let me take him home healthy and sound that I would study hard and become a nurse. I had been accepted into a professional nursing program some years prior, but had decided against it at that stage in my life when the thing I wanted most was to marry Phil and start a family.

During that weekend, Bryan's over-burdened liver suddenly began to function. This was something the liver transplant team had never witnessed. In fact, they were so skeptical they kept the donated liver matched for him on hold in case his own liver stopped functioning again. So we got our miracle. And I wondered if all the praying that our little community church (headed by Reverend Bill Gibson) had been doing collectively for Bryan's recovery had sent some kind of energy through the ether. I wondered if our congregational supplications had actually reached God or a saint, because ten days later, with absolutely no medical intervention, Bryan was given a clean bill of health and discharged from the hospital. The medical team concurred that they too had witnessed a miracle. In fact, they were a little skeptical of this unexplainable rebound in his liver health that they continued to hold his matched liver as long as possible in case it was only a temporary reprieve. Luckily this was not the case and with each passing day, our son continued to progress favorably. We left feeling fortunate, and convinced there was nothing to treat a liver, except for time and rest.

The specialists advised us that Bryan would need a year of rest before returning to school, as he would not have the energy needed to focus on his graduating year of high school. So we found ourselves home, safe and sound, thirty days later, with no protocol for our son other than rest. I couldn't accept this, especially after having seen Bryan so critically ill. I knew there had to be something more my son could do to benefit his health. My friend Andrea Hines recommended Dr. William G. Timmins and the BioHealth Diagnostic Team for a consultation. On their request I sent samples of Bryans saliva and feces. The BioHealth Diagnostic Team clinicians analyzed his samples and then recommended a strict nutritional regimen of organic vegetables, chicken and fish, that would take the stress off of his liver. They also advised against anything from a cow - no milk, no butter, no cheese, and no meat. Bryan was to consume nothing processed or chemically altered with preservatives. Even household cleansers had to be organic and his laundry detergent phosphate free, as chemicals can permeate the skin, the body's largest organ.

Looking back on it all, I wonder why the dairy-*thing* did not register with me until I received the recommendation from the BioHealth Diagnostics. Hindsight is always 20/20. I had always suspected that it was hard on the digestive system, especially since my children had started to have difficulties with dairy as babies. But why did I not accept the fact that it was almost impossible to process and better to avoid? It was only after the BioHealth Diagnostic's advisement that it donned on me that the liver, when burdened, could not handle dairy. The red flag had gone up when Bryan was nine months old. Now it was hitting me right over the head seventeen years later.

We following the dietary regimen recommended by Dr. Timmins, along with another recommendation from Andrea Hines – a video of Dale Figtree. Dale Figtree earned her PhD by leading by example. She used the principle of turning around a life threatening diagnosis of cancer and fighting it with wholesome nutrition. Andrea Hines proved not only a good friend, but also a life-ring for our family in the quest for optimal health. When I feared the worse, Andrea saw the light, the opportunity for change; she stood by us through Bryan's healing process and has left her mark on our family for life. Bryan quickly recovered. His general practitioner saw him that summer, and declared him so fit that he cancelled his follow-up appointment with the liver specialists. He advised Bryan to concentrate on having fun. When Bryan shared with him that his wellness plan was put together by the BioHealth Diagnostic, and that the whole family was following the same strict organic diet, which also omitted alcohol, Bryan's doctor, at the time, suggested to him that the problem was now with 'the mother,' that she was fixated on him and that it would be best if he distanced himself from her and regain his carefree youth. He also assured Bryan that his liver was perfectly fine and that it could handle alcohol and regular food. This was the same doctor who had cancelled my son's follow-up appointment with the liver specialist. Fortunately due to my perseverance in seeking opinions from alternate health specialists Bryan was hearing similar advice from them. The most difficult hurdle is if *one* specialist tells a child what a child wants to hear, he/she may hang-on that one piece of inappropriate advise: a very dangerous scenario for any hormonally-charged teen that wants no set limitations on their social life.

In Canada, it is impossible to see a specialist without a referral from a family doctor. But, our family doctor had taken it upon himself to cancel Bryan's follow-up meeting with the liver specialists that fall, without consulting my husband or me. As our son had been so ill, I wasn't comfortable with this decision. I wanted him to have his appointed check-up with the specialist. So I sent the doctor a letter, explaining how upset I was over the cancelled appointment, and asked if they would see Bryan on my behalf. Thankfully, they were very interested in seeing him, as they wanted to track his progress. When they saw Bryan, they reaffirmed everything that the Mayo Clinic had recommended, and attributed his speedy recovery to his diet. By then, Bryan had put on fifteen pounds. The specialists advised him that excess fat, derived from a poor diet, was dangerous for the liver too. (Amazingly, everything comes back to nutrition!) But Bryan was already increasing his exercise and reintroducing the good foods that Dr. William G. Timmins had recommended.

As Bryan matured, he realized that the cavalier attitude the family doctor had towards holistic health and his mom was dangerous to his personal health. Remember, Bryan had suffered from a liver ailment so severe that he had been placed on a transplant list. For the next two years, our family ate nothing but the diet laid out by the BioHealth Diagnostic team and Dale Figtree's *The Joy of Nutrition*, which recommended a diet of wholesome, unrefined, organic foods, and avoid anything that comes from a cow. Foolishly, I slowly reintroduced dairy to our diet, starting with plain yogurt and a little ice cream. I became violently ill. I vomited, suffered from diarrhea, bloating and sore joints. I had become the next member of my family to suffer from a 'bad cow' experience. As I was concerned about my calcium level and about developing osteoporosis as I aged, I thought I needed dairy. When I shared my concerns with an internist, he laughed and assured me that I would get more calcium from a pill and leafy green vegetables than I ever would from dairy. He recommended that I include vitamin D with my supplements to ensure good calcium absorption. He also advised me that, during the two years that I had eschewed dairy, I had become lactose intolerant, as I had killed the enzyme that helps digest dairy. He said that we are not born with this enzyme, that we develop it as babies, and once it is gone we can't get it back. He told me not to be concerned about it, as I was much better off without dairy. Again, this was another source of professional advice that renounced the goodness of dairy. I found myself accepting that I could not have it, but still buying it for my family members and providing it to guests. It was then that I made good on my promise to God, and enrolled in a nursing program. I wanted to be enlightened in all things healthy, to apply anything that I learned in caring for my family, and to make a career of it. I also accepted that a nutritional diet that restores optimum health is not a *temporary measure*, but a model to live by!

In my Nursing program I learned a lot about health issues that plague various age groups. I studied anatomy, physiology and the various physiological systems, including the endocrine system, and how they interact with each other. I enjoyed my nursing program immensely, and graduated at the top of my class. I attribute this success to my personal search for answers as to why our internal systems inevitably fail. I was a mature student who had experienced the loss of a father due to diabetes and cardiovascular issues. My mother suffers from thyroid and heart conditions, elevated blood sugars, and arthritis. And I have a brother who has had a heart attack. So, I studied each section of my program looking for ways to prevent these conditions from occurring to me or to any member of my family.

Most of what we studied in relation to the treatment of disease was pharmacological. We only touched on nutrition. And the nutrition we did study was the current North American diet, and how poor nutrition leads to cardiovascular disease, diabetes and obesity. But we did not study any real nutritional solutions to the epidemic of North American health conditions that are caused, in part or in whole, by too much bad food. The largest and most difficult core subject was pharmacology. In this course, we were required to study "Pharmaceuticals for Nurses," in its entirety, among other weighty texts. Then we were told that the edition we did study was only the current one, and that a new edition is published every year. Needless to say, this book is more than intimidating!

The end result of my program was that I was fully trained to provide nursing care using conventional health care techniques and therapies. But to learn about alternative or nutritionally based remedies that do not include pharmaceuticals, for my own personal wellness and for my family, I had to do all of the research myself.

We live in a profit driven economy, where the almighty dollar takes precedent over health. Great advertising, funded by large corporations, leads us to believe that we need dairy milk and cheese for strong bones and teeth. Dairy consumption is heavily promoted on publically displayed billboards, in schools, in magazines and in many medical offices. Yet dairy is a known allergen. People crave what they are allergic too, and corporations know this. They also know that dairy has been linked to heart disease and colon cancer, and is the root cause of various other inflammatory diseases, yet they continue to vigorously promote it. My thinking on all of this is that cows belong in the field, and not on the table!

The Raw Live Vegan Lifestyle has you protected!

It is important to keep with you at all times a record of the vitamins that you take, so that if you ever require a prescription, your pharmacist will know of any possible effects these vitamins might have on a prescribed drug. Also keep a current journal that records your food intake, so that your doctor can see if you run the risk of a vitamin or mineral deficiency due to your diet. This is a time for honesty. Let your doctor know if you eat less than two meals a day, or whether your diet is restricted. Perhaps you don't eat dairy or meat products. Your doctor should know this, as this will determine which vitamins and minerals selected to supplement your diet. Also record the amount of coffee and alcohol you consume per day, as these items tend to deplete vitamins or prevent your body from absorbing them properly.

If you follow the Raw Live Vegan program, you will be amazed at how few supplements you will need, as you focus your intake on a raw foods containing most of the essential vitamins and minerals you need. Because they are not cooked, the body more readily absorbs them. A vitamin that is taken by most vegans is vitamin B12, in liquid form, applied under the tongue (sublingually). See Vitamin section for more information on vitamins.

It goes without saying that we do not list meat on our regimen for obvious reasons; nor do we list wheat due to its gluten. Also, note the foods repeatedly appearing in articles and recipes in the Raw Live Vegan program. These foods are also on the Superfoods List.

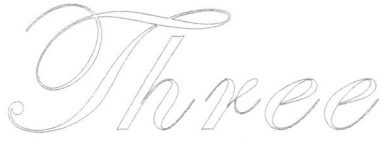

Appliances & Their Benefits

Appliances and Equipment

The First Four are the big ones! But these four can be purchased second hand, refurbished or as a choice gift from a loved one or for self! These four make the raw live vegan lifestyle a breeze!

Blender: Hand held or large jar style. I prefer the Vita Mix Blender, with its two jars. Each jar is geared with a specialty blade for function. One is for dry ingredients, where it turns nuts to flour. The other is for liquids, which will puree ingredients in seconds. Put it on high and it will heat up ready-to-serve. And it's great for soups!

Food Processor: This appliance makes short order of chopping and shredding vegetables, and grinding nuts and seeds. This is definitely a desired appliance on this food plan, when vegetable preparation is the rule of the day. A food processor is a great time saver. I use the robot coupe Blixer #3 – a Christmas present. Some women prefer jewelry, I prefer health-promoting products!

Dehydrator or an oven that allows heat to be maintained at 100-115 degrees F. A dehydrator is a low-temperature oven used to gently dry fruit or prepare raw dishes. It does this by removing the moisture and creating bulkier textures, while maintaining the nutritional integrity of the food. I like my stainless steel D-10, while many of my friends like the Excalibur. The square version of the Dehydrator with many racks is invaluable to making this very healthy transition successful. A dehydrator uses less electricity and costs less than a stove. I currently set my dehydrator up on top of my stove.

Juicer: My favorite juice extractor is the Super Angel. It has two stainless steel augers that extract juice from wheatgrass, leaving the pulp in one tray and the juice in the other. My juice extractor works like a workhorse: it makes nut butter smoother than any other processor on the market. My son has the Breville Juicer and a friend has the Hamilton Beach model. It's important to get a juicer for the sheer health benefits that a juicer provides in breaking down the cell structure, releasing the goodness right into the juice for immediate uptake and little work from your GI tract.

Cutting Board: Wooden boards are best, in a couple of sizes. I use one for fruit and one for vegetables.

Coffee Grinder: Use it for grinding small portions of nuts and spices, which are better for you than coffee – just an opinion.

Mandoline Slicer: This appliance allows you to slice safely and quickly with an assortment of blades and gauges for various thicknesses.

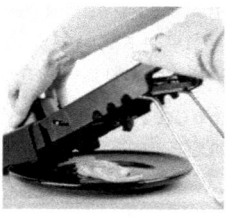

Nut-Milk Bag: This is a fine-mesh bag, usually with a drawstring. It is used for straining juices and nut milks. If you don't have luck finding one in the gourmet section of your kitchen supply centre, try the paint department. I use a fine-mesh bag that was designed for straining paint!

Pastry Bag: This is a great tool. It is used to pipe semi-solid foods through a funnel, thereby creating a decorative touch to your meal presentation.

Sharp Knives: Breakfast, lunch and dinner always feature a fruit or a vegetable, and there is nothing more frustrating than the lack of a good sharp knife.

Colanders: There are a variety of colanders available. I own a few with differing hole sizes. To drain sprouts, or to rinse vegetables or fruit, a large holed colander is fine. Use one with smaller holes for seeds. Use a mesh- style colander to soak cereals and other small grains.

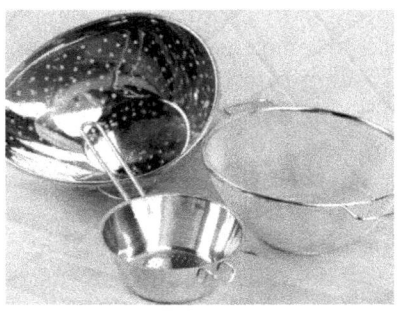

Reamer: I use a hand-held wooden reamer, as it is quick to use, and doesn't take long to clean. Cut a lemon, lime or orange in half, then slightly plunge the reamer into the fruit, and the juice is quickly extracted. Rinse the wooden reamer under the tap and you're done! Reamers come in plastic, stainless steel or wood. There are a variety of sizes too. Remember the glass one with the bowl? They're still out there.

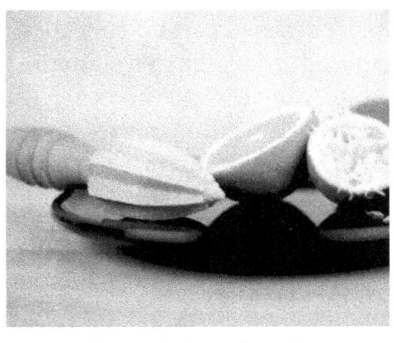

Peeler: There are a variety of hand-held peelers on the market today. With one slice of a peeler, you can make zucchini noodles quickly and easily. Check out the great variety available today at a large supermarket or kitchen store.

Spirooli Slicer: This is a three-in-one gadget that slices, shreds and chops raw vegetables.

Starting Off

To start, if you own a grater, a few large glass containers, a good knife, a stove that will hold heat at a temperature of 100 to 115 degrees Fahrenheit, and a blender you can eat 100% raw and do quite well. When I started, I sprouted in jars. I bought 3 large glass jars with lids, as I knew that I would be buying my first sprouting apparatus some time down the road, and I used them for storing seeds and grains. Also, I thought I would be able to use my oven and cookie sheets, but my oven would not recognize a temperature setting of 100 degrees Fahrenheit. Instead, it automatically rose to 250 degrees Fahrenheit. Most electronic stoves are too new and won't hold a low temperature. But, if your oven will hold a temperature of 100 to 115, then you can dehydrate without having to invest in a dehydrator. Place an independent portable thermostat on the oven rack to ensure that the temperature doesn't exceed 120 degrees Fahrenheit. I place a thermostat in my dehydrator too! For dehydrating purposes, I started with an American Harvest. This is a cheaper version I found at my local hardware store. It was round and had 10 stacks. I used parchment paper, as I could not find round Teflon sheets for it when I needed them. I also cut the mesh bottom out of one of the rings, so I had a spacer ring for dehydrating piecrust. When this worked well, I credited myself with being one of those mothers of invention! If you have the choice, go for a square version. It is much easier to use when making square-shaped crackers and breads. I now own a large stainless steel dehydrator called a D-10. It has 10 shelves with 10 Teflon sheets and 10 mesh screens for nuts. I use all 10 shelves, as I usually have crackers, veggie burgers, and breads going all at the same time!

In terms of affordability, it is cheaper to buy the above equipment than to outfit a traditional kitchen. When you shop the price of a stove, a deep fryer, a grill, a slow cooker, a sandwich maker, a bread maker, a rice cooker and the infinite other products that are available, you will find that the sum cost of the tools required to prepare raw foods is much less. You can swap or sell some of the items that you will no longer use for ones that you need.

Your family will see how dedicated you are to this lifestyle. They will witness its benefits, as they see you regain vitality. They will want you to keep up the momentum, by gifting certain appliances that make your daily chores easier! The more you include and delegate, the more they will see, first hand, what it is you have to work with. A little hint now and then doesn't hurt either!

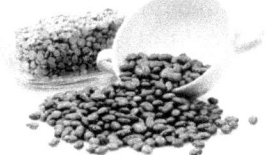

Dehydrating

Dehydration removes moisture from food, the best mode of food preservation. By lowering the moisture content, dehydrating foods effectively keeps bacteria, mold, yeast and natural chemical reactions from attacking the food, while preserving the food's nutrients and enhances the flavor. Vitamin A (beta carotene) and C, carbohydrates, fiber content, potassium, magnesium, selenium, and sodium levels are not altered or lost in dehydration. The same healthy nutrient profile does not exist in canning or chemically enhanced foods with longer shelf lives. Caloric values remain the same but the fat and salt content is reduced. Dehydrated foods are free of pesticides and chemicals.

Dehydrating is the preferred method of preparing some foods. It allows you to cook at a temperature below 120 degrees Fahrenheit, thereby preserving enzymes that are killed at higher temperatures. Dehydrating food dates back to biblical times when it was necessary to preserve food pre-refrigeration era. Food would be dried in the sun or hung to cure. Our generation – with its' savvy food storage technology of preserving foods through refrigeration, freezing, canning, pasteurizing and use of chemical additives – have nearly made dehydrating extinct. Dehydrating is enjoying resurgent health benefits and it involves little time or money! Newcomers to the Raw Live Vegan program will dig their heels in when they realize the time involved in dehydrating a meal or recipe; this is not a problem for the organized person. Know what you want to prepare and adjust your schedule accordingly. The beautiful thing about dehydrating is that you can walk away from it and do other things, but you cannot say the same thing about a stove. Not all meals and recipes require a dehydrator, but for the items that do, like breads and crackers, why not do enough at one time to sustain you a month! Complete meals can be dehydrated and stored safely in the event of a natural disaster when conventional modes of food preparation are not available. Commercially dried foods cost big bucks, we do not know the source of the foods whether they are locally grown or from far away; did the grower use pesticides or chemical additives in the process or use human waste as their fertilizer? By dehydrating your own products you regain control of the end product cheaply! When dehydrating, the idea is to prepare in bulk and to always have something in progress in your dehydrator. I bought one with 10 shelves. I work full-time and manage to have more free time now then when I cooked the conventional way – all thanks to organization. If I want to make bread I realize I have to possibly soak grains nuts and seeds. I do this one-minute chore when I wake up, then I go to work and forget about it. When I get home I mix my ingredients and place in my dehydrator and don't think about it until it is time to flip or take out. I speak the truth here, this mode of food preparation is so easy and fool proof a child can do it. If you add too much liquid, so what, it has to dehydrate longer. The same can't be said about conventional cooking! How many of you can make a perfect pie crust? I couldn't, but I can on this program. The ingredients are simple and they go into a food processor and directly into a pie dish and directly into the dehydrator and voila – perfect delectable pie every time! I prepare 36 nut burgers or 6 racks of crackers at a time, so I always have plenty on hand. I also check my supplies in the freezer to see what I have to prepare next. If your oven can hold a temperature of 100-120 F., then you should certainly use it until you get a dehydrator. But remember, as dehydrating takes time, you might be tying up your primary source of cooking when other family members need it. The other drawback is leaving the house with the oven on for 12 hours, which is not a good idea regardless of the temperature setting.

Your dehydrator has many uses including: servicing as a warming oven, quickly defrosting food, marinating (completed in half the usual time), and reducing sauces. I like it for heating-up a nut butter or chocolate spread to put on my multigrain sweet bread; or for reheating that piece of leftover apple pie that got stashed away in the freezer. Some recipes call for dehydrating at 135 F., but this is due to the low internal temperature and the high fluid content of some ingredients. In this case, the recipe will require a temperature adjustment to below 120 F. as the fluid content evaporates.

Dehydrators have to be watched and monitored for temperature regulation as they are not airtight. I have a temperature setting on my dehydrator, which I back up with a freestanding oven thermometer with a probe. I place it into the dehydrator, and it 'beeps' if the temperature goes higher than the set temperature.

Benefits of Juicing

Juicing improves overall health of everyone, not just those suffering an ailment. It boosts the immune system, increases energy, strengthens bones, clears the skin and lowers the risk of disease. The reason juicing is so beneficial is that most of us in this fast-paced society eat on the run, gobbling our food down quickly with little time to chew it, let alone taste and appreciate it. Juicing does what our slow chewing does even more efficiently: it breaks down the plant cell structure making the various healthy nutrients readily available for quick absorption into our system. What better reasons to juice at least once a day? Selecting a variety of fruits, vegetables and herbs will benefit you in a multitude of ways. Our vitamin section lists their benefits, so you can decide on healthy choices unique to your needs. Always wash foods before juicing, even if they are organic. Because they share shelf space with other produce, chances are that they have been exposed to pesticides.

Juicing with a "Juicer" is a quick way to get your recommended daily servings of fruits, vegetables and water. Yes, fruits and vegetables do contain water! The juicing process removes fiber, and facilitates the rapid absorption of vitamins and nutrients at the cellular level. Juicing oxygenates the cells, due to the abundance of chlorophyll present in fresh fruits and vegetables. This enhances the body's ability to produce hemoglobin, thereby increasing the amount of oxygen that flows to the cells. Processing fruits and vegetables in a "Blender" and adding water makes a thicker drink filled with natural fiber. Fiber is beneficial in cleaning out the GI tract; it also relieves constipation.

Hippocrates stated, "Let food be thy medicine and medicine be thy food." It is important to know whether you have health conditions that are affected by certain food groups. For example, someone with ulcerative colitis should restrict their consumption of citrus fruits, or cruciferous vegetables such as broccoli, cabbage, cauliflower, brussel sprouts or tomatoes. But they can benefit from leafy greens and beets. Keeping this in mind, it's always better to ask someone first before offering them something you have prepared for yourself. It is one thing to "Juice" for your self, but never assume juicing is a healthy alternative for everyone; persons afflicted with certain GI upsets cannot tolerate raw fruit and vegetables. Finally, be aware that although juicing is beneficial to good health, it should never replace whole foods. After all, there is a reason why we have teeth!

For those who are interested in reading further on this topic, I strongly recommend *The Juicing Bible*, by Pat Crocker. This book is full of healthy recipes that benefit the body in general, as well as specific recommendations for juicing for a variety of health conditions.

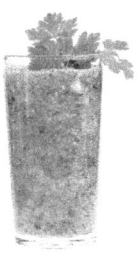

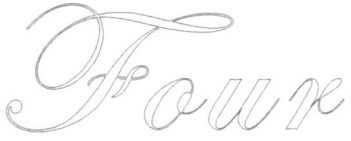

Not Just Your Average Food

Superfoods

Superfoods are foods that contain high amounts of phytonutrients, chemical compounds that occur naturally in plants that may result in extra health benefits. There are many Superfoods, and you have no doubt seen lists citing the top ten. As plant-based nutrition is our life, here at rawlivevegan.com we love to know as many Superfoods as possible. Remember, buy local first and organic is best! A Superfood is not so super when it is sprayed with pesticides. Rinse all vegetables and fruit in pure water and a tincture of wheatgrass juice. To prevent important nutrients from leeching out, do not leave them soaking for long!

Acai berry: is a high-energy berry from the Amazon palm tree found in Brazil. It is high in antioxidants, which prevent premature aging. In fact, the acai berry has the highest concentration of antioxidants compared to other Superfoods. The oxygen radical absorbance capacity or ORAC in acai is off the charts compared to others. The acai berry ORAC score is 610, cranberry is 94, avocado is 19, orange is 18, apple is 43, and blueberry is 53, to name a few. This does not diminish the blueberry or the avocado from being called a Superfood. Understand that these foods also contain other important nutrients making them a Superfood. The acai is also full of amino acids and essential fatty acids. They contain monounsaturated fats (the healthy ones), dietary fiber and phytosterols to help promote cardiovascular and digestive health. Due to its almost perfect essential amino acid complex it is vital to proper muscle contraction and regeneration. Acai berries contain oleic acid, which helps omega-3 permeate the cell membrane, making it suppler. This enables our hormones, neurotransmitters and insulin receptors to function more efficiently. This is important, as we know high insulin levels lead to an inflammatory state causing premature aging. Acai is available in the health food section of your local grocer or at your local health food store.

Avocado: contains monounsaturated fats (a good fat) and vitamin E, two ingredients that help keep your skin nourished. The fat in the avocados helps your body absorb carotenoids, such as lycopene and beta-carotene, from other foods, which may lower your cancer risk.

Barley: is a low glycemic grain that contains both soluble and insoluble fiber. The soluble fiber helps the body metabolize fats, cholesterol and carbohydrates, and lowers blood cholesterol. The insoluble fiber, better known for its roughage, promotes a healthy digestive tract and reduces the risk of cancer. Barley is a good source of niacin. Its B vitamin protects the heart. Barley also contains high levels of vitamin E due to its high concentration of tocotrienols. It provides lignans, which are phytochemicals that function as antioxidants. Women who consume barley are less likely to develop breast cancer.

Beans and Lentils: are an excellent source of high protein and carbohydrate. They are featured on the food pyramid as both protein and vegetable. One cup contains 15 grams of fiber, more than half the recommended daily intake. Due to their slow release into the bloodstream they provide a long-lasting source of sustained energy. Beans and lentils are an excellent source of potassium and help reduce the risk of high blood pressure and stroke. They are also a great source of folic acid, which protects against heart disease by breaking down an amino acid called homocysteine. High levels of homocysteine or inadequate amounts of folic acid triple the risk of birth defects, cancer and coronary disease. Beans and lentils reduce cholesterol, aiding in good heart health. Beans and lentils contain the same potent anti-inflammatory antioxidants, flavonoids and flavonals, and exert antioxidant activity fifty times greater than vitamin E. This protects against oxidative damage to cell membrane lipids, promotes healthy collagen and cartilage, and restores the antioxidant powers of vitamins C and E after they've battled free radicals. Sprouted beans or lentils can be added directly to your salad, on top of your main meals or blended into a dip or soup. Dried beans and lentils should be stored in everyone's pantry.

Berries: Raspberries, blackberries, blueberries and strawberries are packed with disease-fighting phytochemicals that help prevent certain types of cancer. Frozen berries can be enjoyed throughout the calendar year when not in harvest. When frozen at peak ripeness they lose none of their high nutritional level.

Buckwheat: grain comes from the seed of a broad leaf related to the rhubarb plant. Buckwheat is also known as groats or kasha. Buckwheat is beneficial in lowering cholesterol, stabilizing blood sugar levels, preventing diabetes and obesity, and reducing hypertension. Buckwheat is high in zinc, copper and manganese. It is a soluble fibre, which reduces blood glucose levels, a benefit to type II diabetics. It also contains flavonoids, which are known to benefit heart and circulatory health. It is a blood-building food, which supports the circulatory system and helps prevent weakening of blood vessels, as in hemorrhoids and varicose veins.

Cinnamon: Just a quarter of a teaspoon of ground cinnamon added to your food helps lower triglyceride and LDL Cholesterol. Cinnamon is also known to reduce blood sugar levels, a great benefit to type-II diabetics due to the polyphones, which are a natural substance found in plants. Sprinkle it onto your morning groats, in your tea or on your fruit.

Dark Chocolate: is a treat in the true sense of the word. The antioxidant flavonoids in dark chocolate prevent heart disease by reducing inflammation associated with cardiovascular disease. The higher the cocoa content, the better.

Goji berries: are found in Himalaya. They are known for their treatment of high blood sugar, hypertension, malaria, fever and cancer. They are higher in vitamin C than oranges, ounce per ounce. And they contain more beta-carotene than carrots. Goji berries are great on salads, in cereal, or even steeped in tea.

Green Tea: contains polyphenols, which have strong antioxidant properties that reduce the risk of developing certain cancers, liver disease, diabetes and high cholesterol. Green tea has also been known to aid weight loss, so sip away with a touch of cinnamon and now you have *superduperfood*!

Greens Plus: is a powder blend of organic vitamins, essential minerals, live enzymes and antioxidants. One serving, a tablespoon, completes your recommended daily serving of fruits and vegetables. Enjoy *Greens Plus* in your morning shake. See the recipe in recipe section on our site.

Honey, raw: Two teaspoons of buckwheat honey will relieve cough-like symptoms and help with sleep more effectively than dextromethorphan, a cough suppressant drug. Over the counter drugs are not good for anyone. Honey is not always safe in children under 1 year of age.

Kale: belongs to the broccoli, cabbage family. It is high in beta-carotene and vitamins A and C. It also contains sulforphane, a compound that can prevent cancer by helping the body eliminate carcinogens. Also put Kale in salads, in juicer with other fruits and veggies and drink it for its important nutrients. Refer to the recipe section for delicious Kale recipes.

Lemons: are not only good for cleaning around the house, but are good for cleaning the liver. Lemons are high in vitamin C, offer a mini-detox and keep your bowel elimination regular. They are great directly on salads and in water; so treat your self to a gentle detox daily.

Milk Thistle: plant is known as a tonic for the liver due to the active ingredient silymarin. Silymarin is an antioxidant with anti-inflammatory properties that protect the liver. This, of course, depends on the extent of the damage to the liver. Check with your doctor to see if you would benefit. If so, you will need a defined dosage, duration and follow up.

Mushroom: plants are high in vitamin B. They break down carbohydrates into energy-boosting glucose and aid in the normal functioning of the nervous system. Mushrooms boost immune system function, fighting common viruses. They satisfy the appetite due to their "umami," a savory flavor abundant in fattening foods.

Nutmeg: spice is known for treating gastrointestinal disorders by removing gas from digestive tract, which reduces bloating and diarrhea. Nutmeg will relax muscles and soothe circulation. It can be used on many festive treats, vegetable dishes and warm drinks.

Peppers: Red, Yellow and Chili peppers have twice as much vitamin C as green peppers. But green peppers have more vitamin C than oranges and supply more than 100% of the recommended daily dose. Red Peppers have eight times as much beta-carotene as green ones. So get out the salsa and the hummus and start dipping! Chili peppers, known for their heat, are an extraordinary anti-inflammatory, analgesic and anti-cancer food due to their high levels of capsaicinoids, the most common form of which is capsaicin. Capsaicinoids can provide relief to arthritis, headaches and sinus congestion. Most people assume gastric flare up is due to spicy foods where, in fact, the opposite is true. Capsaicin found in chili and jalapeno peppers may actually lead to a cure for certain intestinal diseases. Capsaicin has been found to inhibit the growth of leukemic cells. In South America, where consumption of chili peppers and fiber-rich beans is high, there is a low rate of intestinal, stomach and colon cancer compared to the high levels evidenced in North America. Capsaicin is a known thermogenic agent that helps increase the overall metabolic activity that burns calories and fat and it is all-natural. Use peppers in vegetarian chili, salsa, salads, sauces and dips! Caution, wear gloves when handling jalapeno and chili peppers as their oils will permeate the skin and the heat will become so intense your hands will feel on fire. I speak from personal experience here, WEAR GLOVES when handling hot peppers.

Psyllium: plant acts as a laxative fiber absorbing water and swelling when moving through the digestive tract. You gain the hidden benefits of the high fiber as it lowers cholesterol, controls appetite by offering a felling of fullness, and it helps control diabetes. On the Raw Live Vegan plan we use it as a thickener for sauces. When making a tomato-based sauce, add a tablespoon of psyllium to the recipe and you will be surprised at how less watery it is. Also enjoy psyllium on cereal. Introduce it slowly and, because it is a high soluble fiber, drink plenty of water to avoid bloating and cramping.

Pumpkin Seeds: are high in phytosterols and are renowned for lowering cholesterol and promoting prostate health. They are high in omega-3 and omega-6 and are a good source of phosphorus, magnesium, zinc and iron. Pumpkin seeds are high in fibre and satisfy that desire to crunch. Enjoy a tablespoon on a salad, or alone as a snack! Be aware of the caloric count: 1/4 cup equals 185 calories.

Quinoa: is a supergrain seed containing more protein than most cereal grains. It is considered a complete protein because it contains all eight of the essential amino acids we need for tissue development. Quinoa is higher in calcium, phosphorus, magnesium, potassium, iron, copper, manganese and zinc, and lower in sodium compared with wheat barley or corn. Sprout it and enjoy in salad (see recipe section) or grind to a powder and add to dessert recipes, puddings or breads.

Rhubarb: vegetable is a member of the buckwheat and sorrel family. It contains lindleyin, which is vital to reducing the effects of hot flashes in peri-menopausal women. Research has shown this benefit is derived from estrogen properties found in the root. Rhubarb is high in potassium and vitamin C and an excellent source of fibre. It is known to cause stomach cramps. Caution: Rhubarb root is not recommended for children or pregnant or lactating women.

Shallots: is a member of the onion family and known for its' active ingredient fructo-oligosaccharides. It is a prebiotic that promotes gut health by encouraging the growth and function of good bacteria that live in our digestive tract. Shallots have flavonoids, which play a role in lowering the risk of heart disease and cancer. They are also high in antioxidants. Shallots, unlike their cousins the garlic and the onion, do no cause bad breathe. Eat them raw in salad, soups and spreads. Although onions and garlic fit into this category, shallots are a superior food.

Sprouts: of course, are Superfoods! They are only down this far on the list due to their place in the alphabet! Sprouts contain natural live enzymes - the life force that is lost when cooked. They provide protein, vitamin C and are high in water. Sprouts are much easier to digest than their beans or seeds. They are an excellent source of nutrition, can be grown year round, do not require sun or soil, only water.

Tomatoes: Red tomatoes get their color from lycopene. Lycopene is a fat-soluble antioxidant. Lycopene, part of the beta carotene family, lowers the risk of diabetes, heart disease and a multitude of cancers. Enjoy tomatoes in salads, salsa or tomato sauce recipes.

Turmeric: spice is also known as curcumin and is an active ingredient in curry spice. Turmeric, known to ease aches and inflammation has been used in Eastern civilizations to treat and relieve symptoms of arthritis.

Walnuts: are high in omega-3 (alpha-linolenic acid), containing 2.6 grams per ounce. Who needs fish! Walnuts are also high in antioxidants, amino acids, fibre and protein. They are great chopped and sprinkled over soaked groats with a teaspoon of cinnamon and few chunks of apple.

Quinoa the "Super-Grain"

Quinoa, pronounced (keen-wah), is considered a "super-grain" that is as close to a complete food source as a plant can get, it is though actually a seed. It contains amino acids, enzymes, vitamins and minerals, antioxidants and phytonutrients. It is also high in fiber and is related to the spinach and Swiss chard family, which makes it gluten free!

Not Just Your Average Food

Quinoa is so easily digested for optimal nutrient absorption that it is a must-have for persons afflicted with celiac disease, who have to abstain from other grains. This ancient grain ranges in color from pinks, to browns and reds, to almost black. I mix mine for the colourful effect.

Quinoa is a "super-grain" because it is higher in calcium, phosphorus, magnesium, potassium, iron, copper, manganese and zinc than all other grains. It also contains all nine essential amino acids, which makes it a complete protein. Its high level of magnesium helps relax blood vessels, making it beneficial to people who suffer from high blood pressure and migraines. This amazing grain should be on everybody's table, as it acts as a probiotic that feeds the microflora in your intestines, regulates blood sugar, protects your heart and aids in regularity. And if this isn't enough, higher consumption of this water-soluble fiber, by pre-menopausal women, reduces the risk of breast cancer. The many benefits of this grain explain why it has been around for 5000 years. You can bet it will be around for 5000 years more.

Keep in mind most practicing raw foodies practice 80% raw, and 20% free choice. Quinoa can be sprouted to use in 100% raw recipes; rinse it daily until sprouted, see sprouting technique under article "Sprouting". If you want to cook Quinoa as part of your 80/20% then Quinoa requires rinsing before cooking, due to its bitter coating of saponin. It cooks in only 15 minutes, so it is a great dish to prepare in a hurry. It has a mild, delicate, nutty taste with a light crunch, which lends itself to everything from breakfast to main meal to dessert! Check out our Quinoa salad recipe, or perhaps incorporate it into your soup, for starters. Due to its high level of oil and fat content, Quinoa grains and flour should be stored in glass jars in the refrigerator. Use the grains within a year and the flour within 3 months. When thinking of the food allergies and other conditions that afflict people today, aren't you glad you know about the virtues of Quinoa and can prepare a meal that everybody can enjoy?

For those that enjoy the benefits of the raw live vegan lifestyle, enjoy Quinoa sprouted and eaten in snacks or in salads and sandwiches. Refer to the section in this book on "Superfoods" and discover that Quinoa has its' spot! For more in-depth information check out the following on-line sites:

http://chetday.com/quinoa.html

http://www.bodyecology.com/07/04/12/quinoa_benefits_guide.php

http://lifestyle.iloveindia.com/lounge/benefits-of-quinoa-6494.html

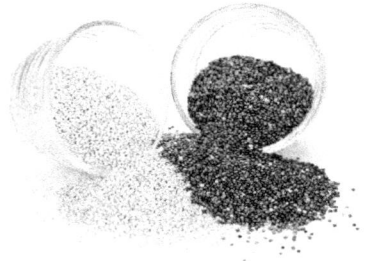

Wheatgrass "A Health Boost"

Green plant cells absorb the sun's energy and store it as chlorophyll. Two ounces of chlorophyll is the equivalent to the total amount of vitamins and minerals found in three pounds of vegetables!

Dr. Max Berner – the inventor of muesli – called chlorophyll 'concentrated sun power.' WG* He said, "Chlorophyll in-

Not Just Your Average Food

creases the function of the heart, affects the vascular system, the intestines, the uterus, and the lungs.... It is therefore a tonic which, considering its stimulating properties, cannot be compared with any other."

Wheatgrass is believed to be approximately 70% crude chlorophyll, making it one of the most potent sources of living chlorophyll available. It also contains 30 enzymes, and is high in calcium, iron, magnesium, phosphorus, potassium, sodium, sulphur, cobalt and zinc. Wheatgrass offers huge benefits to human health. It is a proven blood purifier, liver detoxifier and colon cleanser. (Some health practitioners use wheatgrass in enemas for therapeutic treatments.) It has also been proven to build red blood cells after just 4 to 5 days consumption, which makes it extremely beneficial to those suffering from anemia. The chlorophyll in wheatgrass stimulates healthy tissue cell growth, making it an effective treatment for first and second degree burns. It is used both topically and ingested, as burns can often lead to internal infection. The chlorophyll in wheatgrass also reduces the foul odour associated with burns. The high beta-carotene content in wheatgrass reduces the risk of developing certain types of cancers. Wheatgrass has also been proven to normalize blood pressure and is a great aid in weight control, as it is instantly absorbed into the bloodstream and turns off the appestat in the brain, which causes cravings. It contains no gluten, as it metamorphoses completely into a vegetable with none of the allergic proteins that are common in glutinous grains.

There are many healing centres in the United States where wheatgrass plays a key role in therapies. In the United Kingdom, proponents of wheatgrass offer courses on the benefits of raw, living foods. In one health institute in America, wheatgrass has proved beneficial to patients with terminal illnesses, when conventional therapies failed. In the 1970s, Dr. Ann Wigmore opened the Hippocrates Health Institute, in Boston. There, terminally ill patients were nourished back to health with freshly squeezed wheatgrass. Evidence of the success of wheatgrass in treating serious illnesses has been anecdotal, however, as there have been few, if any, clinical studies.

In the past, scientists who recognized the miraculous benefits of chlorophyll, tried to bottle it. They soon discovered that chlorophyll quickly becomes unstable when packaged. When harvested, wheat grass must be juiced and drank immediately. Wheatgrass may also be consumed in powder form, which keeps for much longer.

I grow my own wheatgrass in my kitchen, hydroponically, and consume two nutritious ounces daily. I have both plastic and ceramic trays and clay pots specifically designed for growing wheatgrass. The clay pots are expensive, so you may opt to soak your seeds on a wire mesh tray that is designed to sit on the lip of the clay tray. Pour water up to the rim of the clay tray; put the wire mesh tray on top of this. The seeds will germinate and send roots down through the rack into the water. There is no more benefit to growing wheatgrass in soil than growing it hydroponically. Hydroponically grown wheatgrass, however, may grow mould. To prevent this, change the water twice a day until the seeds sprout - this is important. Also, spray the seeds with a mix of 3% food-grade hydrogen peroxide. This poses no risk, as the extra oxygen in the hydrogen peroxide evaporates, leaving water to stimulate growth. The only time I had a problem with mould was when I grew wheatgrass on plastic trays. Switching to a wire mesh and glazed ceramic trays proved to be the solution. This method provides better ventilation and I have not experienced mould since then. To benefit from the superior

Not Just Your Average Food

nutrients found in wheat grass, you can purchase Wheat Grass Powder Organic "Triticum Aestivum" (origin: China), from www.starwest-botanicals.com. Or you could sprout and grow your own wheat grass using their gorgeous deluxe wheat grass starter kit, which has easy to follow instructions.

When my wheatgrass grows to a height of 12 to 15 centimetres, I process both grass and roots into a juicer and drink it right away. Including the roots gives the full benefit of this nutritious plant.

Wheatgrass has medicinal value, it is important to consume it slowly and in small amounts. I cannot say enough about the importance of easing wheatgrass into your diet. I recommend starting with a half to one ounce of processed wheatgrass, on an empty stomach. This allows for immediate release of vitamins and minerals into the blood stream. At first, you might feel nauseous due to the immediate reaction wheatgrass has on toxins and stomach mucus. Never exceed four ounces a day; more than this may result in too many toxins being removed from the liver at the same time, causing extreme bouts of nausea. The more wheatgrass you consume, the more nauseous you will feel, so stick to small amounts, always.

For disease prevention, you can make powdered drinks or drink fresh wheatgrass juice as part of a long-term health maintenance program. Unlike fresh, live wheatgrass, its powdered form is not bioactive, but it is nutritionally superior in vitamins and minerals due to its concentrated form. Freshly grown wheatgrass is best if you are attempting to restore your health. Fresh and concentrated wheatgrass powder combined serves as a nutrient and a healer as their benefits overlap. I recommend powdered wheatgrass for travel because it is easier to store.

Some fun facts about wheatgrass: The chlorophyll in wheatgrass makes it an excellent breath freshener, except for the green teeth—just teasing! It can also be used as a face wash. A quarter teaspoon applied topically will clear pimples, remove itch, and make dry skin soft and supple. Regular consumption of wheatgrass boosts the immunities and prevents colds. It also removes toxins, caused by chemical spraying, from fruits and vegetables. If you suspect that the produce you brought home from the market has been sprayed, simply add a tincture of wheatgrass to your vegetable or fruit wash water and quickly soak them before storing. Be aware that soaking for too long may cause valuable nutrients to leach into the water, so be snappy with that produce.

Vitamins, Minerals & Supplements

Vitamins are essential to good health. They are found naturally in fruits and vegetables, and do everything from boosting immune system function to maintaining bone density. Vitamins are either water-soluble or fat-soluble.

Water-soluble vitamins include vitamin B-complexes and vitamin C. Theses vitamins are not stored in our bodies, but are absorbed as needed, and must be consumed every day. Any excess is passed with our urine, making it nearly impossible to overdose. Fat-soluble vitamins include vitamins A, D, E and K. These vitamins are stored in our liver, and do not need to be consumed daily. As excess amounts consumed can be harmful to our renal system, it is important to follow the recommended daily dosage, unless otherwise recommended by a doctor. Although there are countless varieties of vitamin supplements available, we get them, naturally, in whole foods, such as the ones we enjoy on the Raw Live Vegan program. If you eat from the variety of foods recommended on the program, you shall have no problem meeting your daily vitamin requirements without the need for supplements. Ideally, these foods should be Certified Organic and not subjected to irradiation, pesticides and herbicides.

Water Soluble Vitamins

Vitamin B complex is needed for almost every process in our bodies. B vitamins include Thiamin (B1), Riboflavin (B2), Niacin (B3), Adenine (B4), Panthothenic Acid (B5), Pyridoxal Phosphate (B6), Biotin (B7), Folic acid (B9), Cyanocobalamin (B12). Choline is also included in this group even though it is not, technically, a B vitamin.

Thiamin provides our energy stores by converting complex carbohydrates into glucose. Thiamin, Pyridoxal Phosphate and Cyanocobalamin combined regulate our nervous system. Folic Acid prevents neural tube defects in fetuses. Thiamin, Riboflavin, Niacin, and Pyridoxal Phosphate combined aid digestion; without them our bodies would not be able to absorb essential nutrients. The entire group of vitamins, and Choline gives us healthy skin and hair.

It is important to take these vitamins in a complex every day, as they support each other; deficiencies in one B vitamin can cause malfunction of another. Improper preparation and storage may cause leaching, thus reducing their nutritional value.

We all know how little nutrition there is in processed foods, yet the debate over and criticism of healthy, wholesome organic raw food persists. Discussions of vitamin B12 deficiencies, for example, point to vegetarianism as the cause. Some suggest that this vitamin is found in animal protein when, in fact, it actually comes from coenzymes found in and around our mouths. Researcher Dr. Vivian V. Vetrano attributes a vitamin B12 deficiency to a much larger problem, and not to a poor diet. According to Dr. Vetrano, Crohn's and Celiac disease, and other digestive disorders make it difficult for the body to absorb vitamin B12 from natural sources. In these cases injections of vitamin B12 are recommended. Oral supplements are also available. Vegans should eat plenty of healthy raw foods such as grains, nuts, seeds, fruits, vegetables and sea vegetables. My advice to anyone concerned with the myths over vegetarianism, raw food and veganism, is that you should just shake your head at all of that nonsense and move on! See Vitamin Chart for some of the foods containing vitamin B.

Vitamin C is an excellent source of antioxidants. It fights off infection, helps our bodies absorb iron, builds thyroid hormones and collagen, which is an important protein used to make skin, scar tissue, ligaments, tendons and blood vessels. It is also important for maintaining strong teeth and bones. A deficiency in vitamin C causes scurvy. The body does not manufacture vitamin C, nor does it store it, so foods containing this essential vitamin must be consumed daily. The recommended intake of vitamin C is 60 mg/day. Eating a raw diet gives us six times the recommended daily dose of this essential vitamin. See Vitamin Chart for some of the foods containing vitamin C.

Fat Soluble Vitamins

Vitamin A is a carotenoid that supports the immune system, protects us against cancer and heart disease, and helps prevent cataracts. It is found in deep yellow, orange, red and green vegetables and fruits. The recommended daily allowance is 5,000 IU (International Units). Many foods on the Raw Live Vegan program contain Vitamin A. So if you are following the program, you are already aiding your immune system and protecting yourself against disease. See Vitamin Chart for some of the foods containing vitamin A.

Vitamin D supports bone density. Current research suggests that it also prevents some cancers. The main source of vitamin D is sunlight. Ten to fifteen minutes of exposure to sunlight on the arms and face each day is recommended. Those with darker complexions require a bit more time, or a bit more surface exposure as darker skin absorbs vitamin D from the sun more slowly. In the past, the recommended daily intake of vitamin D was 400 IU. Today, due to a lack of sun exposure and the usage of sunscreen, blood work typically shows that most of us are deficient in vitamin D. Recommended daily dosages have also been adjusted upward as research has shown how vital vitamin D is to maintaining good health and fighting off disease. Some recommendations are as high as 2,000 IU a day, depending on the individual need. It is very important not to self diagnose, but rather to undergo blood work, which is a definitive scientific aid in recommending the correct dosage to support good health.

Our ancestors knew the value of the sun and it's ability to prevent disease, to heal, to provide warmth, and so much more. Some ancient cultures worshipped it as a god; others danced to it. Unfortunately, this generation has been brought up to fear the sun, due to the damage too much exposure may cause. Concern over deadly skin cancers has detracted from recognition of its benefits as a natural source of vitamin D – the sunshine vitamin. This article discusses the benefits of natural sunlight, its importance as an essential source of vitamin D, and its contribution to human health.

The current minimum recommended daily dose of vitamin D is 1,000 IU (International Units). In some cases, your doctor might recommend more, depending on your condition. In fact, the National Academy of Sciences Institute of Medicine, in the U.S., suggests that the daily upper limit is 2,000 IU. Whatever the recommended dose, your diet, alone, cannot provide enough vitamin D. You need ample exposure to sunlight and, in many cases, you need to take a daily supplement.

Vitamin D is the only vitamin your body is able to produce naturally. But it can't do it alone; natural sunlight is required. Even though you might spend part of every day outside, you might still not be getting enough sunlight for your body to perform this essential function. You might need to adjust your diet and to supplement.

I get my vitamin D through supplementation topped-off with a little *au-naturel* sunlight; so, set work aside and get outside, reclaim your time in the sun, even if for only 20 minutes. I can't think of a better way to revitalize and re-energize; kind of like plugging into nature's power source! The benefits of vitamin D are numerous. New benefits are being discovered every day. For starters, it helps our body absorb calcium. This is a function we cannot do without this essential vitamin. Calcium promotes bone mineralization, which may prevent or slow the progression of osteoporosis and resulting bone fractures and joint pain.

Sunlight has proven to be a great healer of various skin conditions, such as psoriasis. It has also been proven to alleviate the symptoms of other autoimmune disorders, such as multiple sclerosis and rheumatoid arthritis. Research has shown that vitamin D prevents certain cancers, such as breast, colon and prostate. Further research will, no doubt, increase our knowledge of vitamin D's life- saving capacities.

Natural sunlight can also be mood altering, as it gives your serotonin levels a real boost. Even if you only have a 30-minute break during your workday, try to spend it outside instead of in the staff room. You owe yourself 30 minutes of sunlight each day; this will improve your health and your mood. So, get out there and enjoy the sunshine, you are worth it.

The downsides to vitamin D deficiencies are numerous. Rickets is a disease that afflicts malnourished children in underdeveloped countries. Without sufficient vitamin D, bones become soft. This causes bone deformation and increases the risk of fractures and osteoporosis. Also, when you consider all of the diseases vitamin D alleviates and/or prevents, due to its considerable impact on your immunities, think about what you are leaving yourself open to by not getting enough of this miraculous vitamin. Be aware that it is possible to get too much of a good thing. Vitamin D supplements are fat-soluble; too much can raise blood calcium, resulting in calcification of soft tissues, and cause kidney stones. If you are getting plenty of sunlight, eating foods fortified in vitamin D and taking a supplement, you should consult your doctor to determine whether the supplement is really necessary. A rule of thumb for optimal health has always been 'everything in moderation.' We need to claim our spot in the sunlight and absorb its' wondrous powers, its power to warm and to heal! See Vitamin Chart for some of the foods containing vitamin D.

Vitamin E is an antioxidant that helps stabilize cell membranes and prevent them from breakage. The recommended daily dosage of vitamin E is 30 IU. The Raw Live Vegan diet contains more vitamin E than non-vegetarian's, proof that the Raw Live Vegan program works every time! See Vitamin Chart for some of the foods containing vitamin E.

Vitamin K helps build proteins that allow the blood to clot when we get injured. This vitamin also regulates blood calcium, thereby playing a major role in bone health. The recommended daily dosage is 80 micrograms. Healthy bacteria in your large intestine manufacture vitamin K. Be very aware that antibiotics kill these bacteria and deplete your vitamin K stores. This can upset your fragile electrolyte balance. See Vitamin Chart for some of the foods containing vitamin K.

Vitamins and Their Food Source Chart

Vitamin A	Vitamin B	Vitamin C
apricots	unref. wheat	broccoli
cantaloupes	unref. oats	cantaloupe
carrots	unref. rye	citrus fruits
mango	unref. barley	leafy greens
nectarine	buckwheat	mangos
nori	amaranth	papaya
seaweed veg	coconut	peppers
papaya	flax seed	strawberries
peppers	pumpkin seed	tomatoes
persimmon	sunflower seed	cabbage
plantains	nuts	kale
pumpkin	quinoa	
sweet potatoes	bananas	
tomatoes	legumes/beans	
turnips	leafy greens	
winter squash		

Vitamin D	Vitamin E	Vitamin K
salmon liver	berries	asparagus
mackerel liver	nuts	broccoli
cod liver	raw fruits	cabbage
fortified calcium	sprouted seeds	leafy greens
mushrooms	vegetables	lentils
sunlight	avocados	peas
	olives	pumpkin
		nori
		hijiki
		sea veggies

Minerals

Minerals are elements that are found in soil and water and cannot be created by living things. They include: **calcium, copper, iodine, iron, magnesium, manganese, phosphorous, potassium, selenium, sodium, and zinc.** Plants absorb minerals from the soil. The number and quality of minerals absorbed by plants depends upon the organic matter that it contains. Minerals in farm produce depend on the kinds of fertilizer applied to the soil. Where I live, on Canada's east coast, farmers fertilize their soil with seaweed, which contains iodine. So crops harvested in my local area are high in iodine. Foods recommended in the Raw Live Vegan program are high in all essential minerals.

Calcium is good for bone health. It also eases insomnia and muscle contractions. If you don't get enough calcium from your food, your body will steal it from your bones, leaving them weak and brittle. The recommended daily intake of calcium is 1,000 mg. All fruits, vegetables, nuts, seeds and grains contain calcium. The best fruit sources of this essential mineral are: blackberries, black currants, dates, grapefruit, mulberries, oranges, pomegranate, and prickly pears. See Mineral Chart I for some of the foods containing calcium.

Copper is an essential mineral that helps the body absorb, store and metabolize iron, and form blood cells. A deficiency in copper will leave you prone to anemia. The recommended daily intake of copper is 1.5 - 3 mg. Copper can be found in most fruits, vegetables, nuts, beans, seeds and grains. See Mineral Chart I for some of the foods containing Copper.

Iodine is present in all crops grown in soils fertilized with seaweed, which contains high concentrations of this mineral. Iodine is important to thyroid hormones such as thyroxin, which controls growth, development and metabolism. Iodine also promotes protein synthesis and bone building. Iodine helps regulate the rate of energy production and body weight. Iodine promotes proper growth, and helps promote healthy hair, nails, skin and teeth. Iodine deficiency results in hypothyroidism, goiter and retarded growth.

In developed countries, iodized table salt is found on every dinner table and in most processed products. The recommended daily intake of iodine for adults is 150 micrograms (mcg), and for children, it is 70 - 150 mcg. Seaweed products are part of the daily regimen on the Raw Live Vegan program. This way, we naturally get our recommended daily intake of iodine. Iodine supplements are also available in sea-kelp processed in tablet form. See Mineral Chart I for some of the foods containing Iodine.

Iron is essential for the production of hemoglobin and some proteins and enzymes. It aids the transport of oxygen through the bloodstream and to all parts of our body. It is important for cell growth and differentiation, and for metabolism. It also boosts immunities as it contains antioxidants that protect the body from free radicals. The daily recommended dose for women is 15 mg, for men it is 10 mg, and for children it is 10 to 12 mg. If you are 100% vegan, doubling the recommended daily dose is strongly encouraged. This would mean 30 mg for women, 20 mg for men, and 20 to 24 mg for children every day.

An iron deficiency results in learning disabilities and behavioral problems. It can also result in a deficient immune system, which causes weakness and fatigue. Foods rich in vitamin C, when combined with foods rich in iron, aid in the absorption of this essential mineral. Non-herbal teas containing tannins hinder iron absorption. If your doctor recommends iron as a supplement, and you already take vitamin E, separate the time of day you take these supplements as iron neutralizes this vitamin. See Mineral Chart I for some of the foods containing Iron.

Magnesium is an important mineral needed for clotting blood, activating B vitamins, relaxing nerves and muscles and for energy production. It also aids insulin secretion and function. Magnesium helps the body absorb calcium, Vitamin C and potassium. A magnesium deficiency may result in fatigue, nervousness, insomnia, heart problems, high blood pressure, osteoporosis, muscle weakness and cramps. The daily recommended intake for adults is 310 - 420 mg, and for children it is 130 - 240 mg. See Mineral Chart I for some of the foods containing Magnesium.

Manganese creates enzyme reactions that regulate blood sugar. It also helps healthy bone development, bone metabolism, and calcium absorption. It is important to proper thyroid and sex hormone function, and metabolizes fats and carbohydrates. Recommended daily dosages is 2.0 - 5.0 mg for adults, 2.0 - 3.0 mg for children ages 7 to 10, 1.5 - 2.0 mg for children ages 4 to 6, 1.0 - 1.5 mg for children ages 1 to 3, 0.6 - 1.0 mg for children ages 6 months to 1 year, and 0.3 - 0.6 mg for infants aged 0 to 6 months. See Mineral Chart I for some of the foods containing Manganese.

Phosphorous works in tandem with calcium to aid strong bone and teeth formation, and the formation of nerve cells. Phosphorus is as abundant in the body as calcium. It is prevalent in fruits, vegetables, grains, nuts, and seeds. The recommended daily dose of phosphorous is 700 mg for adults and 500 – 1,250 mg for children. See Mineral Chart II for some of the foods containing Manganese.

Potassium is required for body growth and maintenance. It helps to balance the water between cells and body fluids. Potassium plays an important role in proper heart function. It is also important for the function of the brain and kidneys. It keeps muscle tissue and vital organs in good condition. A deficiency in potassium will result in muscular cramps, twitching and weakness, irregular heartbeat, insomnia, and kidney and lung failure. See Mineral Chart II for some of the foods containing Potassium.

Selenium works with vitamin E as an antioxidant, and is part of several enzymes necessary for the body to function properly. The recommended daily intake is 70 mcg for men, and 55 mcg for women. See Mineral Chart II for some of the foods containing Selenium.

Sodium is found in all fruits and vegetables, and most grains, nuts and seeds. Sodium regulates blood pressure and blood volume. It also regulates the fluid balance in your body, and aids in the proper functioning of muscles and nerves. Passion fruit is naturally high in sodium. Sodium also occurs naturally in vegetables. See Mineral Chart II for some of the foods containing Sodium.

Zinc aids in metabolizing proteins and carbohydrates, aids the immune system and is necessary for wound healing, growth and vision. A severe deficiency results in stunted growth and white spots on the fingernails. The recommended daily intake of zinc is 15 mg for men, 12 mg for women and 10 - 15 mg for children. Vegetarians should consume 50% more, or 23 mg/day for men, 18 mg/day for women and 15 - 23 mg/day for children. See Mineral Chart II for some of the foods containing Zinc.

Minerals and Their Food Source Chart I:

Calcium	Copper	Iodine
Blackberries	Avocado	Iodized salt
Currants	Blackberries	Sea kelp
Dates	Dates	Nori
Grapefruit	Guave	Dulse
Mulberries	Kiwi	Wakami
Oranges	Lychee	arame
Pomegranates	Mango	
Prickly pear	Passion fruit	
Amaranth	Pomegranate	
Bok choy	French beans	
Brussels sprout	Kale	
Butternut squash	Parsnips	
Celery	Peas	
Chinese broccoli	Potatoes	
	Pumpkin	
French beans	Spirulina	
Kale	Winter squash	
Okra	Sweet potato	
Parsnips	Swiss chard	
Swiss chard	Taro	
Turnip	Lima beans	
Almonds	Buckwheat	
Amaranth	Oats	
Brazil nuts	Brazil nuts	
Hazelnuts	Cashews	
Pistachio	Chestnuts	
Sesame seed	Hazelnuts	
	Walnuts	
	Sunflower seeds	

Minerals and Their Food Source Chart I (cont):

Iron	Magnesium	Manganese
Avocado	Avocado	Avocado
Berries	Banana	Banana
Currant	Berries	Berries
Breadfruit	Currants	Dates
Cherries	Breadfruit	Grapefruit
Dates	Cherimoya	Guava
Dried apricots	Dates	Pineapple
Dried figs	Guava	Pomegranate
Grapes/raisins	Kiwi	Amaranth
Kiwi	Passion fruit	Brussels sprout
Lemon	Pomegranate	Butternut squash
Lychee	Prickly pear	
Passion fruit	Watermelon	French beans
Persimmon	Amaranth	Kale
Pomegranate	Artichoke	Leeks
Watermelon	Butternut squash	Lima beans
Bok choy		Okra
Brussels sprout	French beans	Parsnips
Kale	Lima beans	Peas
Leeks	Okra	Potatoes
Butternut squash	Peas	Spirulina
Swiss chard	Spirulina	Winter squash
Sundried tomatoes	Swiss chard	Sweet potato
Nuts, various	Artichoke	Swiss chard
Coconut	Unrefined grains	Taro
Pignolias,	Quinoa	Brown rice
Pumpkin seeds	Almonds	Unrefined grains
Nut butter	Brazil nuts	Coconut
Sesame seeds	Cashews	Hazelnuts
Tahini	Peanuts	Macadamia
Lima/Mung beans	Pine nuts	Pecan
Unrefined grains	Pignolias nut	Pine nuts
Lentils	Pumpkin seed	Pignolias nut
Wild rice		Pumpkin seed

Minerals and Their Food Source Chart II:

Phosphorous	Potassium	Selenium	Sodium	Zinc
Avocado	Avocado	Bananas	Amaranth	Avocado
Currants	Bananas	Breadfruit	Artichoke	Blackberries
Breadfruit	Currants	Guava	Broccoli	Dates
Dates	Breadfruit	Lychee	Beetroot	Loganberries
Guava	Cherimoya	Mango	Bok choy	Pomegranate
Kiwi	Cherries	Passion fruit	Brussels sprout	Raspberries
Lychee	Chinese pear	Pomegranate	Celeriac	Amaranth
Blackberries	Dates	Watermelon	Celery	Asparagus
Passion fruit	Grapefruit	Asparagus	Fennel	Bamboo shoots
Pomegranate	Guava	Brussels sprouts	Kale	Brussels sprout
Amaranth	Kiwi	French beans	Spirulina	Corn
Artichoke	Lychee	Lima beans	Spaghetti squash	French beans
Brussels sprout	Papaya	Mushrooms	Sweet potato	Lima beans
Celeriac	Passion fruit	Parsnips	Swiss chard	Okra
Corn	Pomegranate	Peas	Quinoa	Peas
French beans	Prickly pear	Spirulina	Spelt	Potatoes
Parsnips	Watermelon	Amaranth	Coconut	Pumpkin
Peas	Amaranth	Unrefined Barley	Pumpkin seeds	Spirulina
Potatoes	Bamboo shoots	Unref. Buckwheat		Swiss chard
Pumpkin	Bok choy	Unrefined rye		Buckwheat
Spirulina	Butternut squash	Brazil nuts		Oats
Taro	French beans	Cashews		Rye
Unrefined grains	Lima beans	Coconut		Cashews
Brazil nuts	Parsnips			Pine nuts
Cashews	Potatoes			Pignolias nuts
Pine nuts	Pumpkin			Pumpkin seeds
Pignolia seeds	Spirulina			Sunflower seeds
Pumpkin seeds	Sweet potatoes			
Sunflower seeds	Swiss chard			
	Unrefined grains			
	Almonds			
	Chestnuts			
	Coconut			
	Pistachios			
	Pumpkin seeds			
	Sunflower seeds			

Omega-3

Omega-3 referred to as 'food for the brain,' is an essential fatty acid that benefits our overall health, and should be consumed daily. As the body can't produce it, we must obtain omega-3 from food. Omega-3 is critical to brain function and to normal growth and development.

Omega-3 acts as an anti-inflammatory that helps reduce blood clotting, which lowers the risk of heart attacks. It is also known to help prevent depression and slow the progression of Alzheimer's. It helps prevent Parkinson's disease, and reduces the risk of breast, colon and prostate cancer. Studies are currently underway on the effect Omega-3 has on asthma, dysmenorrhea, eczema, lupus, pre-eclampsia, nephritic syndrome, schizophrenia, stroke prevention, ulcerative colitis and ADHD.

Salmon and sardines are the two most familiar sources of omega-3. Recent discoveries of heavy metals found in these fish have been cause for concern. As heavy metals are toxic, decreased consumption of these and other fish species has been recommended, especially for pregnant women. Nevertheless, we can still get our marine-based omega-3 in supplement form, as supplements are purified through a process that removes these toxins. You can also take a combination of plant and marine-based omega-3. But you should be aware of the differences.

Plants and marine life contain different types of polyunsaturated fatty acids. Marine sourced omega-3 contains EPA (eicosapentaenoic acid) and DHA (docosahexaenoic acid) fatty acids. Plant-based omega-3 contains ALA (alpha- linolenic acid) fatty acid. The body can't make any of these acids, but it can convert ALA into DHA and EPA. According to Canadian dieticians, this process only happens if we avoid trans and saturated fats and limit our intake of other oils such as safflower, sunflower and corn oil. Also, even in the process of conversion, we still need to be concerned about whether we are getting enough omega-3 from plant-based sources. Marine life is jam packed with omega-3, whereas plant life offers comparatively smaller amounts.

Farmed Atlantic salmon contains 2,153 mg of omega-3 per gram. Hemp oil, on the other hand, offers 1,000 mg of omega-3 per 1 tablespoon. Ground Flax contains 900 mg of omega-3 per tablespoon, and 1 tablespoon of walnuts offers 750 mg of omega-3. Knowing that the current recommended daily amount is 500 mg per day, any one of the above foods supply more than we need. All of these plant-based foods are on the Raw Live Vegan program, so if you are following our recommended regimen, you are more than covered.

As there are no heavy metals in marine-based supplements, and if taking them doesn't pose a health risk, then it seems logical, for now, to continue doing so until we know, for sure, how much EPA and DHA is produced in the conversion of plant-based ALA. It is also important to remain open-minded and to keep current on new findings on this important subject. But before taking any supplements, consult your family doctor. Omega-3 can pose health risks to someone taking a blood thinner such as warfarin, to diabetics and to those with a risk of bleeding such as hemophiliacs.

Omega-3 and Their Food Sources

Chia seeds	Tuna	Krill
Salmon	Algae	Nut oils
Sea vegetables	Flaxseed oil	Sardines
Hemp oil	Halibut	

Vitamins and minerals are found in all foods before they are cooked. But when we cook them, we lose the water, fat-soluble vitamins and enzymes needed to transport minerals into the cells. This leaves the body in a de-mineralized state. But our body, being a miraculous and dynamic structure, compensates by withdrawing minerals from our bones. Most people supplement their diets with vitamins and minerals, and there are vast arrays out there. As we all have independent needs, due to our own current health condition, it is important to discuss supplements with your doctor. Carefully select the best vitamin supplement regime for you to follow. Provide a list of your supplements for your doctor to review with your annual blood work. This will help determine whether your supplement regimen needs adjusting.

It is important to keep with you at all times a record of the vitamins you take, so that, if an emergency requires you to take a prescription, the prescribing physician will know of any possible negative contraindications. You should also keep a current journal to record your food intake, so your doctor can see if you run the risk of a vitamin or mineral deficiency due to your diet. Food journaling is a time for honesty. Let your doctor know if you eat less than two meals a day, or whether your diet is restricted. Perhaps you don't eat dairy or meat products. Your doctor should know this, as this will determine which vitamins and minerals are selected to supplement your diet. Also record the amount of coffee and alcohol that you consume per day, as these items tend to deplete vitamins or prevent your body from absorbing them properly.

If you follow the Raw Live Vegan program you will be amazed at how few supplements you will require. Focusing on your intake of *raw* foods containing most of the needed essential vitamins and minerals, allows for better absorption of nutrients (because they are not cooked). A vitamin that I do I recommend taking daily, however, is vitamin B12, in liquid form.

It goes without saying that we do not list meat on our regimen for obvious reasons; nor do we list wheat due to its gluten. Also, note the foods appearing repeatedly in articles and recipes on the Raw Live Vegan program are also foods you will see on the Superfoods List.

Prebiotics & Probiotics

"Oh my goodness let's simplify these two!"

Prebiotics and probiotics help restore the balance of bacteria in your digestive tract. Probiotics are beneficial bacteria that line your GI tract. They are found in fermented foods such as sauerkraut, miso, tamari, shoyu, and tempeh. They are also found in pickled ginger, yogurt (made with lactobacillus or bifidobacterium) and breast milk. A good probiotic supplement source is acidophilus.

Prebiotics feed beneficial bacteria in your gut, and create a healthy environment for natural flora to thrive. They help moderate cholesterol and triglyceride levels, thus reducing the risk of atherosclerosis (hardening of the arteries) by 30%. Prebiotics also boost immunities, by boosting white blood cells and killer T cells. They come from carbohydrate fibers, called oligosaccharides, which are not digestible, but remain in the digestive tract and stimulate the growth of beneficial bacteria. Sources of oligosaccharides/prebiotics include herbs, such as chicory or burdock, and dandelion root. Prebiotics are also found in fruits, such as bananas and apples, legumes and whole grains. Yogurt, made with bifidobacteria, contains oligosaccharides. Fructo-oligosaccharides may be taken as a supplement or added to food. Yacan syrup is a good example of a fructo-oligosaccharide (review the section on Sweeteners). Prebiotics are also found in certain sweet vegetables, such as onions, garlic, asparagus, leeks and Jerusalem artichokes, and raw apple cider vinegar and breast milk.

Healing From The Inside Out!

Healing from the inside out takes time and patience. It must start with a thorough physical examination appropriate to your age and sex, so your doctor can rule out any serious health conditions. Once you have ruled out any environmental issues and your doctor gives you the go-ahead to embrace optimal health through optimal nutrition, you will begin to feel results almost immediately. Among them are healthy weight management and increased energy. Be patient, as total optimal health – from the inside out – takes a good seven years. If you are currently on medication do not take yourself off of them. Instead, work with your doctor as you embark on this journey. Have regular check-ups more than once a year. Your doctor will be more than interested in charting your progress if you show a real desire to improve your health. He or she may also adjust and likely eliminate medications as your health improves.

Most diseases can be avoided by eating real food. Some of the preventable diseases and poor-health conditions include cancer, diabetes, obesity, and inflammatory disorders such as arthritis and gout. Some of these latter conditions can even be reversed through good nutrition. Even dementia can be avoided, as it has been linked to poor nutrition and environment. You can revitalize yourself by eating raw, organic, live food without supplementation. Refer to our section on Vitamin & Mineral Supplements to find-out which foods contain which nutrients and how minerals get into our food. We don't need supplements from a bottle when they are naturally available in food! Be sure to buy organic, as toxins in foods fertilized with chemicals and sprayed with pesticides impede the body's ability to absorb nutrients. They also damage our immune system, never mind vital organs.

Become familiar with our section on "Superfoods" and make sure you eat the rainbow. By eating the rainbow, I mean a colourful variety of fruits and vegetable, from the darkest of greens – such as broccoli and kale – to the bluest of blues – such as blueberries. A variety of fruits, vegetables, whole grains, legumes, nuts, seeds, oils, vinegars, spices and yes even our sweeteners all play key roles in promoting optimal health. Become intimately familiar with our allowable food lists. Another great reference for the newcomer is "Raw Food 101." All other articles relating to food, such as Antioxidants, Omega-3, and Wheatgrass are to your benefit. Understanding the science behind the foods will keep you motivated. Adopting this lifestyle is a process of learning and doing. Knowledge is power.

Working with a doctor is important to your success, especially if you have food allergies or an upset GI tract. This doesn't mean you won't be able to adopt this optimal food program or adapt it to your needs. But you may have to heal a condition first and start slowly.

Your current body chemistry is a product of your personal food choices. You choose what you eat and what you put into your body. At any given moment you choose health or disease. Disease stems from consuming foods that are inadequate and of no nutritional value. The way to turn this around is to eat the foods on this program that are capable of restoring your health. People confuse prescription drugs as a cure. Drugs may support some diseases - leprosy for example. However, if you are using a statin drug to lower cholesterol for example, then this is not a cure, but rather a means of managing symptoms. Statin drugs may produce better lab readings in blood work, but proper nutrition *actually* solves the problem by lowering cholesterol and negating the need for a statin drug! If you are on a statin drug and are not familiar with CoQ10, ask your doctor if this is a supplement you should consider taking. Never ever take yourself off of a prescribed drug instantly. Let your doctor gauge your prescribed drug and titrate the dose lower as your condition improves.

Become familiar with the Raw Live Vegan program. Acquire the necessary foods and transition at a rate that is comfortable for you. There are no gimmicks in this program. It simply offers good information on clean food and its importance in restoring health. As we consume food that is raw, live and organic our organs sing.

Fortifying the body with nutritious food is like turning-on the lights. We acquire vitality and enhanced energy as our metabolic rate increases. The accumulated toxins in our system from unhealthy eating are purged, and our skin glows.

We are what we eat, so be mindful of what you put into your mouth. Do not take for granted the good results you enjoy in the short term, as your work has just begun. This program is not a fad, nor does it offer a quick fix. It takes seven years of this new way of eating to achieve total rejuvenation. This is a lifestyle for longevity. In this book, we discuss environmental issues to create awareness, so you can form your own opinion and decide what is important to you. You, alone, are responsible for your health. We cannot change the world, but we can change ourselves.

Health is wealth, so take your health seriously. Aim for longevity. And remember, longevity comes from a system that is well nourished over the long term. First, make an appointment with a doctor or nutritional expert, and get started!

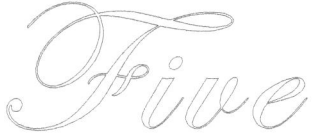

Taking Food Knowledge To The Next Level

The Evolution of Gluten in the Name of Science!

Gluten comes from grass related grains such as wheat, barley, rye, kamut and spelt. It is the consumption of these products that can affect the health of humans and pets alike. Gluten intolerance is as old as time itself, but why is it becoming more common? Is it because the tools in diagnosing gluten intolerance have evolved or has the wheat itself evolved (thanks to genetic modification)? Science collides with Mother Nature in their aim to mass-produce food rapidly and cheaply. Wheat is the number one crop in the world, which nourishes humans and animals alike. Wheat is a popular crop based on its' diverse uses. Science steps in to protect the crop by genetically altering it to make it pest and pathogen resistant and give it the ability to grow in any climate. It is these gluten proteins "glutenin" combined with gliadin in wheat, or secalin in rye or with horedin in barley which are the elastic proteins known as prolamins that have been altered genetically to yield a high-molecular-weight glutenin, which improves bread-making qualities. Imagine that, a better glue! It's no big mystery that by genetically altering wheat to increase its' gluten has also increased the number cases of gluten intolerance. Genetic modification impacts our environment, economy, ecology and ultimately our health! Even some canines have gone gluten-free, largely due to the increased ill effects from the gluten in commercialized dog foods. Dog owners deem their health a priority, and say no to GMOs!

Gluten is a protein composite, not a protein in itself. Gluten is insoluble in water, creating bulk to the diet. Gluten gives bread products that chewing satisfaction we have come to crave. When we think of cravings we think of varying food consistencies such as chewy, crunchy, creamy and smooth. Recently substantial studies suggest our bodies may not tolerate and digest gluten as well as we assumed. It is believed more people suffer the effects of gluten intolerance albeit the symptoms differ in range from slight to incapacitating.

Abstaining from Gluten does not equate to inferior nutrition. To enhance the nutritional profile of your gluten-free lifestyle consider non-grass members such as buckwheat and quinoa. These alternative grains offer fibre, thiamine, riboflavin, niacin, folate and iron. The protein found in these "pseudo-cereals" are higher in arginine and histidine than in their gluten counterparts. Quinoa and buckwheat are essential for optimal health in infants and children.

Those who enjoy a raw live vegan lifestyle comprised of raw plant-based organic nutrition in its' purest form benefit exponentially! Science may offer up its' so-called *healthy* alternative in a processed version for your convenience. The commercialization and processing of these gluten-free products offer an inferior nutritional profile. Consumers have to be vigilant in knowing the source of gluten-free products; cross-contamination with gluten products occurs at the packaging level if a company also packages grains containing gluten. Vegans face a similar risk of contracting e-coli in a restaurant that does not practice good hygiene with food preparation by not thoroughly cleaning produce, or by using the same cutting board as to prepare meat.

It would be relatively simple for the gluten intolerant person to maintain optimal health if they *only* had to avoid particular grass-like grains containing offensive gluten. Unfortunately this is not quite so easy. Consumer foods have evolved to what I consider unrecognizable products with a list of ingredients so long and distorted from actual food itself. Gluten is used in sauces, flavourings, flavour-enhancers and even as a binder or filler in vitamins and supplements, which is why I always recommend vitamins in veggie-cap capsules. At the risk of being morbid, let it be known that vitamins with gluten binders have been found to be completely intact postmortem. Need I be more specific in trying to tell you gluten is difficult for the body to break down and absorb? Gluten has been found in more than just grains; it is now being added to dairy products in the form of casein, soy and corn! Remember science sings the virtues of gluten as a binder, and a "filler," and a form of elasticity that makes bread making wonderful; wonderful at what cost to your health, though?

Ignoring symptoms of gluten intolerance can lead to leaky gut, anemia, hormonal imbalance, bowel cancer, hypothyroidism, diabetes type II, pancreatic insufficiencies, neurological dysfunction, osteoporosis, musculo-skeletal problems, as well as a host of other health issues. The symptoms vary from mild to debilitating, and are typically exacerbated by emotional trauma and stress. Many of the symptoms associated with gluten intolerance are the same symptoms exhibited by people with Crohn's disease, chronic fatigue, iron deficiency, irritable bowel syndrome and intestinal infections. There can be a crossover between gluten intolerance and any of the aforementioned conditions, and made worse by unsuitable food choices.

Gluten Intolerance Symptoms:
- Weight loss or weight gain.
- Nutritional deficiencies due to mal-absorption of vitamins and minerals.
- Gastro-intestinal problems such as bloating, pain, gas, constipation and diarrhea.
- Fat in the stools due to poor digestion.
- Aching joints.
- Depression.
- Eczema/Rash.
- Head aches/Migraines.
- Exhaustion.
- Irritability and mood swings.
- Infertility, irregular menses, and miscarriage.
- Cramps, tingling and numbness.
- Slow infant and child growth.
- Candida.
- Decline in dental health.

Everyday, people assume they can tolerant gluten as long as they are not allergic to wheat; they assume they have an in-depth knowledge of what agrees with them and what does not. Gluten intolerance can be best explained in three distinct groups; celiac disease, non-celiac gluten sensitivity, and wheat allergy symptoms. There are silent celiac disease symptoms that can create havoc and irreparable damage to your GI tract.

1. Celiac Disease occurs when gluten triggers your immune system to overreact with strong and unusual antibodies. Celiac Disease wears down and destroys the villi lining your digestive tract. Villi are the tiny finger-like hairs that absorb nutrients from the foods passing through the GI tract. Villi transport the absorbed nutrients into our blood stream. If villi are damaged

we suffer the effects of nutrient mal-absorption, which is evident in blood work. The only way to diagnose Celiac disease is through blood testing for high levels of anti-tissue transglutaminase antibodies (tTGA). If a blood test proves positive for celiac a biopsy of the small intestine during endoscopy is performed. A narrow tube called endoscope is inserted through the mouth and stomach into the small intestine. Amazingly, one can have celiac disease and not have a wheat allergy! With the high prevalence of GMO food products in the marketplace, one would think that testing for gluten intolerance would be part of an annual check-up for every person and every pet.

2. Non-Celiac Gluten Sensitivity is difficult to diagnose, as those tested for celiac would come back as negative. The only way to diagnose non-celiac gluten sensitivity is to eliminate gluten from the diet and monitor symptoms.

3. Wheat Allergy Symptoms are different from Celiac Disease and Non-Celiac Gluten Sensitivity. A wheat allergy is a histamine (inflammatory) response to wheat that manifests in symptoms varying from hives to stomach pain. One can have a wheat allergy and not have celiac disease!

I associate gluten with "glue" – hard to metabolize! For most persons going gluten-free equates to optimal weight. To eat a gluten-free diet even if you are *not* gluten intolerant is a choice, a choice no different then choosing to eat dairy-free or vegan.

If at this point you decide to eat dairy-free for a prolonged period of time and have not previously been lactose intolerant you will be. Prolonged abstinence from dairy kills the enzyme that aids in the processing of lactose. We are not born with this enzyme, but we "develop" it as a child when introduced to dairy. Although, the enzyme required to digest lactose does not develop in every person. Further, as an adult we cannot develop the enzyme a second time after it has been lost.

Personally speaking my health soared when I abstained from gluten, meat and dairy! I developed www.rawlivevegan.com to show you that you can make everything from scratch without the additives. Sauces and condiments such as gravy, ketchup, mayonnaise and vegetable dressings can be made with merely a few organic ingredients. All of your food can be prepared from scratch, while you still maintain a full-time career. The foods suggested on the raw live vegan program energize and revitalize so you have plenty of energy for nutritional food prep at the end and/or start of each day. Persons consuming processed, genetically modified convenience foods find themselves lethargic, overweight, forgetful and hormonally imbalanced. My cravings and health issues disappeared with this change in choice of a raw live vegan lifestyle. We are living in a time when food is not just food.

http://www.icyou.com/topics/diseases-conditions/celiac-disease-and-gi-research-part-2+

http://amazingglutenfree.com/2010/07/31/dr-fasano-leds-stem-cell-research-for-celiacsgluten-free/

http://www.celiac.com/articles/1131/1/Refractory-Celiac-Disease-Responds-to-Stem-Cell-Transplant/Page1.html

The Importance of pH Balance

If we compare our bodies to a finely carved sculpture, a good nutritional foundation would be like a piece of fine Italian marble. We select the best nutritional regimen possible and we shape it with exercise. Next, we smooth the rough edges by adding a special blend of hormones according to our personal needs. For some, this will mean bio-identical hormones to correct a diagnosed hormonal imbalance. For others, it might mean the addition of nutritional supplements or certain foods from specific food groups. The final touch, which gives the artwork its aesthetic appeal, is making sure that our nutritional choices lend to a healthy pH balance.

Balance in nutrition, hormones, and especially pH are key to optimal health. When we discuss pH balance we are not talking about the acid in our stomachs. We are talking about the body fluids and tissues that are measured at the end-stage of digestion, or how our body filters the foods we eat. The pH scale ranges from 0 to 14, 7.0 being neutral. A pH greater than 7.0 is alkaline (basic), and a pH lower then 7.0 is leaning toward acid. The rare conditions brought on by pH levels at the two extremes of the spectrum are called acidosis and alkalosis. These conditions are rare but everyone has a tipping point. Due to our current North American diet, it is common for North Americans to fall into a slight state of acidosis more than a slight state of alkalosis. People can be in a state of mild acidosis for years without realizing it is the root of their health problems. Mild to full blown acidosis will manifest itself with the following symptoms: heart related issues with onset cardiovascular damage, including the constriction of blood vessels and the reduction of oxygen, leading to high blood pressure; weight gain, obesity, and diabetes; hormonal imbalance, low energy and chronic fatigue; immune deficiency; bladder and kidney conditions, including kidney stones and gout; premature aging; candida, and yeast/fungal overgrowth; stalled metabolism and slow digestion, resulting in slow elimination, and a consequent build-up of toxins in the digestive system; joint pain; aching muscles and lactic acid buildup.

The body is truly an amazing organism, comprised of 70% water. This is a gift, as water has a perfectly neutral pH of 7.0. This is the best reason I know for grabbing a glass and drinking plain water throughout the day. Your body has a natural ability to remove acid from its system. When you have too much acid build-up, your body steals minerals such as calcium, magnesium, sodium and potassium from your vital organs and bones, to neutralize this acid and safely eliminate it. But, your body can only pull so much from vital organs and bone before it falls into a state of acidosis. This state of mild acidosis can go on for years, contributing to what we have accepted as being part of the normal aging process.

The opposite condition of alkalosis is extremely rare. It is usually caused by high altitude, a lack of oxygen, liver or lung disease, or salicylate poisoning. The symptoms of alkalosis are hand tremors; light-headedness; muscle twitching; nausea; vomiting; numbness or tingling in the face or extremities. Again, alkalosis is rare and not induced through bad nutrition.

I find the prevalence of acidosis unacceptable. As a nurse, with a focus on disease prevention as opposed to seeking remedies in pharmaceuticals, I suggest we look at how to avoid them entirely. The answer is found in our diet. We consume far too many acid-forming foods, and put ourselves into a state of mild acidosis for too long. The results have been that many of us exhibit one or more symptoms associated from highly acidic food choices. It is time to reassess our diet.

The typical North American diet is high in acid-producing animal products such as meat, eggs and dairy products, and far too low in alkaline-producing foods such fresh vegetables and ripe fruit. Remember, I said fresh and ripe, as they become more acidic when cooked. We also consume acid-producing beverages, such as coffee and soft drinks, and eat processed foods such as white flour, refined sugar, processed meats and frozen entrees. This pH imbalance is self-induced through the consumption of acid-producing foods that leave us in a less than optimal state of health. How did we get there? Simple: our hormones take a pounding through improper nutrition and stress. Hormone levels can be determined through blood work.

If we are in a sickly state of acidosis, physical activity should be minimal. Healthy cells thrive in an oxygen-rich state and an alkaline base. In an acidic environment, cells mutate at an accelerated rate, creating free radical damage, and possibly contributing to cancerous mutations.

Testing pH is very easy with pH test strips, available at a local pharmacy. The timing for the most accurate results is the same as it is when testing for sugars - one hour before a meal or two hours following a meal. You can test by dipping a pH strip into your urine, to see if it is excreting toxic acids from your body. Your pH should not be below 6.0. If it is, it is too acidic. Your urinary pH may range from between 6.0 - 6.5 in the morning and 6.5 - 7.0 in the evening. Throughout the day normal pH ranges fluctuate between 6.0 -7.5, which is considered optimal. You can also test your saliva for pH balance. Saliva is the liquid generated beneath your tongue. Simply dip the strip into it, and hope it is not below 6.5. If it is, this means you are leaning toward an acidic state. You can also gain an accurate reading through blood work, which ideally should read 7.36.

Do not attempt to test your pH by test stripping the food you consume. A case in point: a pH test strip on raw meat will register alkaline; a pH test strip on a lemon slice will register acidic. But after they are digested, the body fluids show pH levels that are the reverse. It is in the digestion of these foods and the end products they produce after assimilation that we register the body tissue and fluids for pH levels. If your urine and saliva are both below 6.5, then you need to make an immediate nutritional and supplement intervention by consuming more foods that are alkaline.

Creating the perfect balance is easy - simply follow the Raw Live Vegan program. All raw vegetables and vine-ripened fruits are alkaline. Foods not on the program, and that contribute to our high acidity levels, include eggs, dairy, meat, caffeine, alcohol, soda pop, processed foods, and refined flour and sugars. Knowing that the body tries to maintain a perfect pH balance, and that it will steal from our bones and vital organs to do this, the onus is on us to aid our system through the best possible nutrition. If you suffer from any of the aforementioned conditions related to acidosis, then you already know the cause. The cause is none other than your food choices and how you prepare them for consumption. I know this sounds harsh, but you alone can turn this situation around and help your loved ones to do so as well.

Think of the pH scale in simplified terms: High Alkaline, Moderate Alkaline, Low Alkaline, Neutral, Low Acidic, Moderate Acidic, and High Acidic. To achieve the optimal state of Neutral toward slight Alkaline, 80% of one's daily food choices should come from the Neutral to High Alkaline ranges of the pH charts. You can still choose 20% of your desired food items from the below Neutral range of the pH charts, but know that these choices are less than desirable as they are acid forming. No wonder why persons suffer ill health when we witness 80% or more of their food choices coming from the acid forming choices!

Taking Food Knowledge To The Next Level

Food pH Levels Charts

Sweetener pH

High Alkaline	Stevia
Mod Alkaline	
Low Alkaline	Raw Honey, Br. Rice Syrup, Dr. Bronners Barley Malt
Neutral	Sucanat
Low Acidic	Barley, Cornmeal, Rye
Mod Acidic	Processed Maple Syrup#1, Proc. Molasses, Fructose, Proc. Fructose
High Acidic	Cane Sugar, Beet Sugar
Acid Forming	Artificial Sweeteners

Fruit pH

High Alkaline	Lemons, Watermelon, Cantaloupe, Limes, Mangoes, Dried Dates, Dried Figs, Melons, Papaya
Mod Alkaline	Dates, Figs, Apples, Grapes, Avocado, Kiwi, Bananas, Currants, Gooseberries, Raisins, Grapes, Grapefruit, Guavas, Kumquats, Nectarines, Passion Fruit, Peaches, Pears, Persimmons, Pineapple, Quince, Raisins, Tamarind, Tangerines, Umeboshi, Plums
Low Alkaline	Oranges, Carob, Cherries, Pomegranate, Sun-dried, Olives, Raspberries, Sour Grapes, Strawberries
Neutral	
Low Acidic	Processed, Olives, Blueberries, Cranberries, Plums, Prunes
Mod Acidic	
High Acidic	
Acid Forming	

Oil pH

High Alkaline	
Mod Alkaline	
Low Alkaline	
Neutral	Almond, Avocado, Canola, Castor, Coconut, Corn, Margarine, Olive, Safflower, Sesame, Soy, Sunflower
Low Acidic	
Mod Acidic	
High Acidic	
Acid Forming	

Vegetable and Bean pH

High Alkaline	Alfalfa Grass, Kelp, Barley Grass, Kudzu root, Parsley, Kamut Grass, Wheat Grass, Juices from Veg., Seaweed, Watercress, Wheat Grass
Mod Alkaline	Squash, Asparagus, Carrot, Celery, Swiss Chard, Dandelion Greens, Endive, Endive, Escarole, Leaf lettuces, Pumpkin, Spinach, Peas, Rutabaga
Low Alkaline	Brussel Sprouts, Bamboo Shoots, Sweet Corn, Beets, Broccoli, Cauliflower, Cabbage, Cauliflower, Collards, Cucumber, Daikon, Eggplant, Ginger, Kale, Kohlrabi, Leeks, Iceburg Lettuce, Mustard Greens, Okra, Parsnip, Peppers, Pickles, Sweet Potato, Radish, Swiss Chard, Taro, Turnip, Waterchestnut, Green Bean, Lima Bean, Snap Bean, Sprouted Beans
Neutral	Artichoke, Artichokes, Horseradish, Mushrooms, Onions, Rhubarb, Sauerkraut, Tomato, Soy Products
Low Acidic	Adzuki, Blk Bean, Broad Bean, Garbanzo, Kidney, Lentils, Navy, Pinto, Red, White
Mod Acidic	
High Acidic	
Acid Forming	

Meat and Animal Product pH

High Alkaline	Breast Milk
Mod Alkaline	
Low Alkaline	
Neutral	Butter unsalted, Raw milk, Raw cream, Eggs, Goats Milk, Lactobacillus acidophilus, Lactobacillus bifidus, Cow's whey, Goat's whey, Yogurt plain
Low Acidic	Butter salted, Processed Butter, Mild cheese, Medium cheese, Crumbly cheese, Cows homogenized milk, Processed cream, Custard, Egg whites, Goat's Milk Homog., Lamb fat, Chicken fat, Fish fat
Mod Acidic	Fish with fins, Sharp cheddar, Custard with sugar, Shellfish, Whole eggs fried, Yogurt sweetened, Beef fat, Pork fat
High Acidic	Bear, Beef, Chicken, Deer, Goat, Lamb, Pheasant, Pork, Rabbit, Turkey, Custard with preservative
Acid Forming	

Starch pH

High Alkaline	
Mod Alkaline	Arrowroot Flour
Low Alkaline	Potatoes
Neutral	Essene Bread, Granola
Low Acidic	Bran, Millet, Sprouted Millet, Unrefined rye crackers, Unrefined rice crackers, Wholegrain pasta, Popcorn plain
Mod Acidic	Corn, Oat, Rice, Buckwheat hot cereal, Cream of Wheat, Oatmeal hot, Refined crackers, Whole grain with honey, Popcorn with butter, Tapioca
High Acidic	Wheat, Refined Cereals with sugar, Refined Pasta with sugar
Acid Forming	

Nut pH

High Alkaline	
Mod Alkaline	
Low Alkaline	Almonds, Coconut fresh
Neutral	Chestnuts
Low Acidic	Brazil, Cashew, Coconut dried, Filberts, Macadamia, Pecan, Pistachio, Walnut
Mod Acidic	Peanut
High Acidic	
Acid Forming	

Seed pH

High Alkaline	
Mod Alkaline	Alfalfa sprouted, Chia sprouted
Low Alkaline	Radish sprouted
Neutral	Sesame seed
Low Acidic	Pumpkin seed, Sunflower seed
Mod Acidic	Wheat germ seed
High Acidic	
Acid Forming	

Grain pH

High Alkaline	
Mod Alkaline	
Low Alkaline	
Neutral	Amaranth, Millet, Quinoa
Low Acidic	Barley, Cornmeal, Rye
Mod Acidic	Basmati Rice, Brown Rice, Buckwheat, Oats
High Acidic	Bleached Wheat, White Rice, Spelt, Wheat
Acid Forming	

Condiment pH

High Alkaline	Organic Cayenne Pepper
Mod Alkaline	Gelatin with Veg/Fruit, Chives, Marjoram, Dr. Bronner's Mineral Boullion, Vegetable Salt, Bay Leaves
Low Alkaline	Basil, Celery Seed, Dill, Oregano, Rosemary, Sage, Tarragon, Ketchup Homemade, Miso, Sea Salt, Bio-Salt, Caraway Seed, Cloves, Coriander, Cumin Seed, Curry Powder, Fennel Seed, Ginger, Paprika, Tamari, Vanilla Extract, Apple Cider Vinegar with Mother, Sweet Brown Rice Vinegar
Neutral	Mayonnaise homemade, Org. Processed Salt, Soy Sauce, Anise, Cinnamon, Brewer's Yeast, Nutritional Yeast
Low Acidic	Plain Gelatin, Natural Mustard, Mustard Dried, Nutmeg
Mod Acidic	Sugared Gelatin, Ketchup sugared, Mayonnaise sugared, Mustard Refined Artificially Flavoured with Preservative, Soy Sauce Processed with Sugar
High Acidic	Table Salt, Vinegar White Processed
Acid Forming	

Miscellaneous pH

High Alkaline	
Mod Alkaline	
Low Alkaline	
Neutral	
Low Acidic	
Mod Acidic	Cigarette Pure Tobacco
High Acidic	Non Organic Cosmetics, Prescription Drugs, Cigarette Chemically Processed Tobacco, Pure Chewing Tobacco
Acid Forming	Chemically Processed Chewing Tobacco with Sugar

Beverage pH

High Alkaline	*Alkalizing Water, Fresh Juice from Vegetables, Parsley Juice, Wheatgrass Juice, Fresh Squeezed Juice from Fruit
Mod Alkaline	Carrot Juice, Herbal Teas from Leaves, Alfalfa Juice, Clover Tea, Mint tea, Sage Juice
Low Alkaline	Beet Juice, Raspberry Herbal Tea, Ginseng, Herbal Teas from Root, Ginger Tea, Spearmint Tea
Neutral	Comfrey Tea, Non chlorinated/nonfluoridated water.
Low Acidic	Coffee Substitute Chicory, Natural Fruit Juice
Mod Acidic	Wine, Organic Coffee Beans, Fruit Juice with Sugar
High Acidic	Liquor, Beer, Decaffeinated Coffee, Caffeinated Drinks, Carbonated Drinks, Soft Drinks with Artificial Sweetener, Black Tea
Acid Forming	

*Alkalizing water a specialty item found at most upscale specialty health food stores.

The Theory of Food Combining

Food combining, also known as trophology, is based on a theory that suggests as different food groups digest at different rates, it is best to combine compatible foods for good digestion and optimal nutrient absorption. Food combining is usually recommended to relieve gastrointestinal problems or to isolate or eliminate suspected allergies. Following a strict regimen designed and managed by your doctor is the safest way to introduce food combining into your diet. Personally, I would only follow such a rigid program if I was experiencing gastrointestinal (GI) upset and wanted to find the root cause, and only if my doctor recommended it.

There are a number of possible reasons for GI upset. These include flu, contaminated or spoiled food, allergies, and food sensitivities. Allergies and food sensitivities can occur when certain foods are combined. But it is important to rule out other factors before pointing toward a food allergy or sensitivity as the possible cause and seeking medical assistance. A sensible approach to nutrition is always best.

Strong advocates of food combining aim for optimal food absorption with minimal gastrointestinal symptoms. They design their diets around the time it takes each food group to digest, and combine accordingly. For example, most fruits digest in one hour (except melons which digest in 15 minutes). In general, vegetables digest in 1 1/2 to 2 hours, but some vegetables move more slowly through the digestive tract. Carbohydrates and starches take 2 to 3 hours to digest, and proteins digest in 3 hours. According to the food combining theory, proteins, vegetables and fats go together; carbohydrates, starches and vegetables go together; proteins and fats should be separated from carbohydrates and starches; and fruit should be eaten alone. This method would surely be of benefit of those eating cooked foods, which have lost their living enzymes during preparation. The body generally works harder to access the digestive enzymes needed to break down these foods – the biggest culprit of slowed digestion is meat and dairy. However, if one consumes enzyme-rich raw foods, these foods digest easily on their own, making food combining unnecessary. On the Raw Live Vegan program, proteins and carbohydrates are all plant-based, which makes them all the same food group in terms of the time it takes them to digest.

Although there is a mass movement attesting to the benefits of food combining, many of the assumptions used to justify this program are not supported by biological and medical science. In fact, there is currently very little research-based evidence to support this theory. I for one can appreciate the theory, especially for those who ingest meat or dairy as they take a long time to digest. I also can see the importance if one was trying to figure out a specific allergen that causes GI upset. There are a variety of sources with differing opinions on the benefits and degree of strictness required when following food-combining principles. Some combine food to address specific health complaints. Others believe when foods are raw, and when they are organic and exclude dairy, eggs, and meat, and when the protein and carbohydrates come from plant-based sources (such as fruits, vegetables, mushrooms, nuts, beans, and seeds) that it is difficult to differentiate between specific groups. For plant-based foods are both protein and carbohydrate; and in some cases fruit and vegetables are too! Also, in some cases their digestive times merge.

Keep in mind digestion starts in the mouth with mastication (salivation), and food being broken-down by salivary juices, which are more alkali so as to protect teeth enamel. Digestion progresses as food moves into the acidic stomach and then into the more alkaline environment of the small intestine.

Medically, food combining has successfully treated thousands with such food related conditions as acid reflux, gas emissions, and Irritable Bowel Syndrome (IBS). But for some, these conditions may have been temporary and may possibly have cleared up without resorting to food combining.

For most conditions, the best food plan is a raw food diet spread over three meals a day. Three meals a day is pretty standard and seems to work best in today's busy society. Your GI tract needs time to digest food, so three hours between meals is optimal even if you follow food combining.

Vegetables are the one food group that combines well with all others, making them a great snack whenever hunger strikes. For the most part, fruit is eaten alone either twenty minutes before a meal or two hours after. Fruit is acidic and passes through the acidic stomach more quickly that other foods. Also, on the raw food program, some of the fruits and nuts are mixed, which works against food combining principals. More important than science, common sense says to listen to your body and avoid foods that cause indigestion or discomfort. Personally, I do not experience any discomfort when I combine different food groups in my raw food regimen. I enjoy fruit in my morning *Greens Plus* shake, which also includes natural plant-based proteins (Vega Complete Whole Food Health Optimizer), vegetables (Spirulina), and carbohydrates (flax meal). I feel that this program has enough of its own rules without having to worry about food combining. Be assured that your weight loss will be permanent on a raw food plan, and all of your nutritional needs will be covered as long as you stick to the basics.

It has been shown that most diseases affect those with a high acidic pH balance. This is where the Raw Live Vegan program is superior, as it recommends eating citrus fruits that move through the acidic stomach quickly. It recommends vegetables, nuts, and legumes, which are more alkaline. It also stresses the avoidance of meat and dairy – both require the body to become more acidic to aid in their digestion. Thankfully, Raw Live Vegan foods are gaining momentum, and restaurants that offer 'Raw Food' as a healthy option are opening up across our nation and throughout Europe.

Fasting

Our bodies are constantly being bombarded with toxins. They are found in the air we breathe, the water we drink, the cosmetics we apply to our skin, the laundry detergent and cleaning supplies we use, in the foods we eat and in their packaging. The main form of control we have of limiting exposure to toxins comes in our selection of food. The amount of toxins we ingest directly from food depends upon what we eat and drink, as well as how it is grown, packaged and prepared. As we digest our food it is broken-down into carbohydrates, proteins, fats, vitamins, minerals and toxins. All of this passes through our permeable intestinal wall, enters our bloodstream, and is transported throughout our body. Our system absorbs the nutrients it needs and removes toxins. Some toxins are eliminated through respiration, through our skin and through our feces. But some toxins accumulate in our kidneys and liver. When these organs become saturated, excess toxins are stored in our fat cells. Fasting helps our bodies eliminate toxins. But fasting is only recommended for those who are in optimal health, and preferably under a doctor's guidance.

Our kidneys, liver, lungs, lymph nodes and skin work in harmony to remove toxins from our bodies. Although our kidneys' main task is to keep our body's pH level in balance, they also play an active role in filtering toxins from what we eat and drink. When we consume a high acidic diet of coffee, meat, processed drinks, soda pop, alcohol and sugar, our kidneys must work hard to alkalize our system. Adding toxins into the equation means the kidneys have the even harder task of breaking-down and passing on the toxins to the liver.

The liver is our body's main detoxifier. By consuming a diet replete with foods from the "Foods to Avoid" list (such as coffee, alcohol, and meat), we demand the liver to work overtime. A toxic diet combined with exposure to toxins in our environment and household products adds up to an overloaded liver. When the burden of filtering toxins is too cumbersome for the liver to handle, it passes on toxins to our fat cells. To protect the vital organs from harm, fat cells encapsulate and store toxins. When existing fat cells can't endure any more toxins, the body forms more fat cells.

During inhalation our lungs breathe in rich oxygen, absorb it through our alveoli, pass it on to our bloodstream and transport it throughout our bodies. Our lungs then collect carbon dioxide from our blood and expel it with exhalation. Deep breathing, particularly aerobic exercise, is vital for optimal lung health. It goes without saying that smog and cigarette smoke make the lungs' job much more difficult than they are naturally designed to perform.

The lymph glands, appendix, spleen, thymus, and tonsils are organs we are lead to believe we can 'live without,' as they have historically been removed when even slight problems arise. But these organs perform very important roles in detoxing the body as well as immunity. Because they swell up in a state of toxicity, their condition can also serve as a measure of whether our bodies are overloaded with toxins. When our tonsils or appendix are removed, the second line of defense becomes our immune system. And when our immune system is weakened, people tend to resort to pharmaceuticals to mask symptoms. In this case, removing toxins is even more vital to prevent organ failure.

Signs of toxic build-up include acne, rash, or boils. When we try to cover acne or a rash with make-up, the pores become clogged. Our skin is our largest organ and it needs to breathe. As it is porous, it absorbs and releases toxins. Rather than sealing in toxins with make-up, ask what have we been exposed to that caused the reaction in the first place. Listlessness, general fatigue, mental fogginess, insomnia and headaches are a few signs of toxicity. When we are experiencing any of these symptoms, it might be time to fast.

When planning a fast, choose a day when you know your energy demands will be minimal. Optimally this would be on a day-off from work and one when you have the house to yourself. Moodiness and lethargy are common while on a fast. You may even experience a mild breakout as your body expels toxins. Everyone reacts differently, which is why it is prudent to choose a day when there are few demands for your energy.

For a liquid fast, start the day with a drink of water and lemon before breakfast. For breakfast include only organic fruit, *Greens Plus*, spirulina and purified water. For lunch and supper include juiced organic vegetables, wheat grass and sprouts. In between breakfast, lunch and supper enjoy herbal teas, wheat grass juice or purified water with lemon. In colder climates juices can be warmed to 118 degrees Fahrenheit. In hot climates enjoy them chilled according to your personal preference. Feelings of queasiness can be subdued by adding cayenne pepper or ginger and cucumber to your tea or water.

On the day after your fast, breakfast should also be liquid. A fast should be broken the next day starting with water and lemon, followed by your regular breakfast shake, and then a regular light lunch and supper.

After completing a few one-day Raw Live Vegan fasts you will be able to predict how you will respond to it in the future. Personally, I fast only when my body suggests the need; I'm prompted to cleanse when I feel sluggish or if a vacation or holiday compromises my Raw Live Vegan lifestyle. Listen to your body. If your body is running efficiently, why fast? We are all unique. Some people enjoy a fast and experience immediate benefits; they may even plan ahead for the next one. Complimentary and supportive practices during fasting might include a massage, meditation, listening to great music, or reading a great book. Regardless of how you spend your day of fasting, at the end of it you feel clean, energized and invigorated.

Even though we should spend our day relaxing and meditating, fasting in the way of the Raw Live Vegan provides you with energy and a feeling of being nutritionally satisfied. It nourishes vital organs while encouraging them to detoxify. On the other hand, a strict "Water Fast" will leave you feeling weak and listless. It is tough on your system, as it gets right down to the business of eliminating toxins from the body – and at a rapid rate. Again, quick elimination of toxins forces your organs to work overtime and may also cause a sort of healing crisis. If too many toxins are released in a short period of time you will feel depleted of energy – physically and mentally. Water is not sufficient for any fast. In order to do a "Water Fast" you must be in optimal health before starting. Then and only then consider the possibility of implementing a fast one-day a week. Listen to your body!

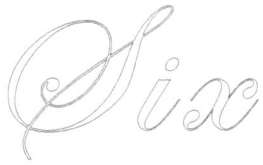

Three Keys To Success

Hormonal Imbalance Through the Lifespan

Thanks to the many authors for shedding light on hormone-related health issues and reaffirming my sanity that what I was going through was very real.

Abnormal hormone levels are often missed in our annual check-ups, as we can appear to be healthy when we really have underlying illness that could be hormone-related. Hormonal imbalance can happen at any age, even as early as adolescence. Normal hormone levels play a major role in healthy aging. This is why it is so important to recognize symptoms and seek professional advice. Aside from aging, factors that influence our hormone levels include pregnancy, as well as exposure to toxins in our environment, household products and the foods we eat.

Healthy, happy hormones need to be addressed at every stage of life. I strongly urge young men and women to have their hormone panels done early in life, so they can track changes as they age. As a baseline, women should have a hormone profile done in their early thirties, or before starting to have children – whichever comes first. Doing so enables the comparison of hormonal levels after childbirth to determine if there are irregularities indicating the need for treatment. Follow-up should continue as they age. Men can wait until in their forties to have hormone panels done, as this is when they typically experience a reduction of testosterone levels. Although rare, extenuating circumstances may point to the need to investigate earlier.

Your hormone profiles are uniquely yours, and at any point shall be compared to previous tests rather than some chart citing what is normal for your age. Regular hormone testing helps you track and compare hormonal changes over time. It could also help you and your physician determine the root cause of any number of health issues.

There are two ways to test hormones for profiling: the first is a saliva test; the second is a serum test that requires blood work. The problem with either of these tests is that you could send three different samples to three different laboratories and get three different readings. There is much debate over which is the most accurate, serum or saliva. It comes down to the physicians' competence level in reading results and in handling content in the lab. I did both serum and saliva testing; both indicated estrogen dominant with progesterone depletion. If you choose to undergo the saliva test be sure the lab you send your sample to is proficient in this area. Testing procedures must be performed to professional gold standards. Also, a certified medical or laboratory director should be available to consult with your physician on their findings. Some physicians are more comfortable with serum testing and are competent in reading results. For females, either test should be taken over a three-month period at different intervals throughout the menstrual cycle. I was tested on the 10th and 17th day of my cycle. Every woman's cycle length varies: some are 28 days, some are longer or shorter; but day 1 of a cycle is always the first day of menstrual flow.

Women are often treated for several possible conditions before any thought is given to hormonal imbalance. The reason for this is simple: most general practitioners know about a multitude of conditions, but endocrinologists have a better understanding of the impact of hormones on body function and health. In Canada it is difficult to have access to an endocrinologist without the required referral from a general practitioner; and if the primary care physician doesn't see a need for you to do so, chances are you won't be referred. If you are suffering with chronic weight-gain than the thyroid may be dysfunctional. Even a modest increase of thyroid stimulating hormone (TSH) can cause weight gain. In this case, your doctor should fill-out a blood work requisition to test your thyroid hormones – checking levels of TSH, Free T3 and Free T4, as well as the antibody levels.

The indexes of standard allowances for vitals and serum levels have been altered over the years to meet the statistics of our demographic population. This means, the more people that are over-weight the higher the 'average' weight is in our population. Standard index charts are adjusted to match the 'normal' and 'healthy' weight to the weight of the 'majority' of the population. Like the height to weight ratio, measurements of vitals and blood serum levels in tested populations have changed. So, 'acceptable ranges' in height to weight ratio, blood sugar levels, body mass index, cholesterol and blood pressure have all been adjusted. Acceptable hormone ranges have also been adjusted! The reason for changes of the standard 'healthy' measurements is that if indexes were not adjusted, for example the height to weight ratio, everyone would be charted as over weight. The primary reason people are over weight is largely due to what the population is consuming. Since the introduction of steroids, food additives, and GMOs to our food chain the average body weight of people has increased, and their health has decreased.

According to Dr. Natasha Turner in her book *The Hormone Diet*, an optimal TSH measurement should be less than 2.0, and not the currently 'acceptable' 4.7 reported by most labs. T3 and T4 should be in the middle of your lab's reference range.

The key to regaining optimal health is to ensure your hormones are balanced. Some of us go through changes in life with little or no effect. Others suffer from a broad range of conditions that may be attributed to hormone imbalance. Some of the symptoms of hormonal imbalance include fatigue, weight gain, excessive weight loss, loss of muscle mass, low libido and/or emotional strain. Having your hormone panels checked helps you identify whether your hormones are in balance or if not, which ones need to support. I use a topical cream of bio-identical plant-based progesterone. This has increased my energy, permitting me to exercise; in turn, my metabolism has increased. I started taking these hormones at 52 years of age, but only after finding a doctor who was willing to discuss my issues with me and consider that they were not a part of the normal aging process. I emphasize the use of bio-identical hormones because they are natural. They are also tailored to a patient's specific hormonal requirements.

An alternative to natural bio-identical hormones is a hormone supplement, such as *Premarin*, which is made with the urine of pregnant mares. This is a drug that may be taken for ten years only and then it must be stopped cold turkey. The pharmaceutical company Wyeth will say their trade drug *Premarin* is natural; of course, horse urine is natural... for a horse. There are other ways to balance hormones. For some, it may require adjusting food intake. For others it may require a prescription. *Premarin* is ingested, which means that it travels through your GI tract. It is also mass-produced in pill form and not formulated for your own specific hormonal requirements. Worst of all is the number of side effects attributed to this drug, including nausea, fluid retention, migraine headache, breast tenderness, stroke, heart attack, blood clots, cardiovascular disease, and breast cancer. Bio-identical hormones are applied in a cream and absorbed through the skin directly into the blood stream, or in an easily swallowed pill form. The downside of taking a natural hormone supplement, or any hormone supplement for that matter, is that it sends a signal to your body telling it to either cease or reduce its natural production of that specific hormone. This means the body becomes dependant upon a hormone replacement. Until the root cause for the body's inability to produce the hormone is address the body will continue to require a supplemental form. Even slow, progressive reduction in dosage does not allow your natural hormone production to resume to its former rate. The body will produce hormones in a balanced fashion when the body itself is in balance.

Keeping this in mind, if you are considering hormone replacement therapy that it's important to be certain you actually *need* hormone replacement as opposed to an adjustment in diet or lifestyle. I use hormone replacement therapy because my blood serum tests showed definitively that I needed it. And I always prefer the natural supplement to anything artificial. This will require ongoing annual blood work to keep an eye on my hormone levels too – an easy routine I am willing to adhere to.

If your tests show you could benefit from hormone replacement, do yourself a favor by taking control over what you are being prescribed. You also need to decide whether you and your doctor are on the same page when it comes to natural treatments such as bio-identical hormones. Initially, I addressed all of my symptoms through whole, low calorie foods, and exercise even though I was so fatigued. And I still gained five pounds every year starting in my mid-40s! I went from the bottom of my weight range for my age and height to the top. Yet my general practitioner was not willing to help me until my waist circumference exceeded 34 inches or I hit the top of the weight range for my age and height. I did not want this trend to continue as I reached full-blown menopause. I soon discovered that the problem was not with my doctor, but rather with my expectations of him. Had I been clear about the direction I wanted my health to go, and asked more specific questions, he may have been able to refer me to someone else, or tell me straight up that this was not his field of expertise. The problem was that I wasn't really sure what to ask. I made the assumption that since a prescription was required, any doctor could write it. However, I came to realize there was something wrong. I also knew I wasn't happy with my doctor's recommendations, which boiled down to: come to see me when you're a real wreck. This is when I started to investigate on my own and found many of my problems were related to hormone imbalance. For me, the prescribed topical bio-identical hormones, a healthy raw food diet and exercise helped me achieve the optimum health I enjoy today.

Additional contributing factors to hormonal imbalance are petrochemicals added to foods and other products, such as every-day household cleaners and cosmetics. Petrochemicals, also known as xenoestrogens, imitate the effects of estrogen on our bodies, thereby interfering with normal hormone function. This is especially devastating to men as it negatively impacts testosterone levels and fertility. Petrochemicals pervade our environment. They contaminate our water, air and soil. Animals and plants making up our food supply – and that depend on good clean air, soil and water –

have become more toxic and less nutritious over the years due to exposure to petrochemicals. Petrochemicals are also found in plastics, dry cleaning chemicals, personal hygiene products and the pesticides that are used to prevent disease and infestation in the fruits, vegetables, grains, nuts and seeds that we eat. Add all of this to the chemical fertilizers used to super-sized crops and hormone additives used with livestock and there's no mystery as to why so many people are so sick.

Our government encourages commercial farmers to provide more meat and produce for a growing population. Science permits farmers to do this at a profit by providing the means to genetically alter our food. Further processing of foods with additives and refined sugars has also contributed to unhealthy hormonal imbalance. Government and science have given little or no considerations to the impact chemical laden foods have on our health. Thankfully, new knowledge in this area has caused a growing shift toward organic foods. It is interesting to note, however, the rules and regulations for the certification of organic farmers are more difficult than for commercial farmers; the latter of whom continue to use petrochemical fertilizers and growth hormones despite inadequate study of the impact they have on human health.

The key to regaining your health will be through hormonal balance, a healthy diet of whole raw foods, and increased physical activity. Keeping a daily journal of what you eat, the time of day you eat it, as well as any physical activity you do, the quantity and quality of your sleep, and how you feel are also very important. And don't forget to list any supplements or medications you take. All aspects of your daily regimen are pertinent to your optimal health. Before consulting your doctor on health issues, particularly if you suspect they may be hormone related, ask yourself a number of probing questions. Be honest when answering them. Jot them down in your journal and take them with you to your next doctor's appointment.

Questions for women to consider

Possible signs of hormonal imbalance, peri-menopause or menopause:

- Do you experience fatigue?
- Do you have elevated cholesterol?
- Do you have allergies?
- Do you have asthma?
- Do you have recurring infections?
- Are you under severe emotional stress?
- Do you suffer from chronic pain or physical stress?
- Do you have low blood pressure?
- Do you have a low resting pulse rate (fewer than 70 beats per minute)?
- When you rise quickly do you feel light headed?
- Do you have difficulty losing weight?
- Do you have cold hands and feet?
- Are you sensitive to cold?
- Do you have difficulty concentrating?
- Do you have poor short-term memory?
- Do you feel depressed?
- Do you have premenstrual mood swings?

Questions for men to consider

Signs and symptoms of hormonal imbalance or andropause:

- Do you experience fatigue?
- Do you lack initiative?
- Are you less assertive than you once were?
- Have you experienced a decline in your sense of well-being?
- Do you feel depressed?
- Are you frequently irritable?
- Has your self-confidence declined?
- Do you find it difficult to set goals?
- Do you have a difficult time making decisions?
- Do you have gallbladder problems?
- Do you have enlarged breasts?
- •Have you experienced a decline in your mental sharpness?
- Have your stamina and endurance decreased?
- Have you lost muscle mass, strength, or tone?
- Have you gained body fat around your waist?
- Do you have elevated cholesterol?
- Has your libido decreased?
- Have you lost interest in sex?
- Is it difficult to obtain or maintain an erection?
- Have you lost your morning erection?
- Do you have sleep apnea?

If you suffer from a number of the above conditions you may possibly be experiencing hormonal imbalance. My suggestion is to keep a detailed journal for one month. Record everything you feel and experience in the areas of eating, rest, physical activity, mood and feelings. And then take your journal with you when you consult with your doctor. Suggest to your doctor that you would like to have your hormones tested. (I used the serum test as our local lab was experienced in this method and it was my doctors preferred hormone testing method.) Your lab results may offer an indication as to why you feel the way you do. Find a physician knowledgeable in dietary nutrition as well as hormones. To find a knowledgeable doctor, I conducted a search on the Internet for "compounding pharmacy" and discovered a list of local compounding pharmacies and doctors. Another avenue is to enlist a doctor with the designation MD and ND, a doctor knowledgeable in both natural and pharmaceutical based medicine. In addition, follow a healthy diet with whole raw foods such as those recommended in the Raw Live Vegan program. As you feel your energy returning, add exercise to your regimen, thereby balancing the three essential components to optimal health. The end result will be balanced hormones, vitality, weight management, true health and a happier you.

Benefits of Exercise

Today's busy, technologically driven society has all but made exercise obsolete for the masses. We drive everywhere, due to urban sprawl. "Those of us who are privileged enough to live in the country drive even more. And when we aren't in our cars, we are seated at our desks, in front of our computers, corresponding on-line with colleagues: sharing documents, social networking or placing an order to be packaged and shipped to our door."

We live by a day-planner. And we work long hours in order to squeeze every last task into our jam-packed lives. We worry about getting ahead, making ends meet, putting the kids through college, saving for retirement, and leave little or no time for exercise. Then we find ourselves ready to retire and we don't even have the strength or stamina to enjoy it.

Before it's too late, recognize the lack of exercise contributes to premature aging. If you are on medications, chances are this can be attributed to poor lifestyle choices. After a hard day's work, we feel entitled to eat what we want and when we want, and to unwind using the various relaxants or stimulants that are readily available, including junk food, fast food, caffeine, alcohol and nicotine. And we usually consume these while social networking on our computers or sitting in front of the TV. This type of lifestyle raises cortisol levels, creating stress and adding to food cravings, nervous tension and sleepless nights. If this is your lifestyle, then you are on a proverbial treadmill conducive to premature aging.

Without question, moderate daily exercise improves health. It controls weight, moderates blood pressure, builds healthy bone, and keeps your heart healthy by decreasing cholesterol. Eating more foods from the Raw Live Vegan plan, which are more alkaline, will help to prevent arthritis and osteoporosis. It also reduces stress, which is the most common complaint voiced by members of the workforce. Reducing stress helps us concentrate and become more organized. When you notice how exercising helps you to move systematically through your daily tasks with focus and energy, perhaps you will see the value in scheduling workout time into your day-planner.

Medicine cannot replace what healthy eating and moderate exercise do for your body. Exercise burns calories and increases muscle mass, which in turn increases metabolism because muscles contain fat burning enzymes. The resulting weight loss decreases blood sugar and the risk of developing Type II diabetes. Excess weight is also the most common factor in high blood pressure, as well as wear and tear on your joints. Assess your own lifestyle, with your doctor's guidance, to see what changes can be made for a successful health outcome. It could be something as simple as doing your own household chores, taking the stairs at work or parking a little further away from the grocery store when you are running errands. Get a dog that suits your lifestyle and your home; take him for walks and enjoy the park.

It's important to choose physical activities you enjoy. Find a buddy with similar goals and interests and keep each other motivated and on track. But whatever exercise routine you choose, remember to avoid being over-enthusiastic. If you set the bar so high that you burn yourself out, you will become discouraged and begin to hate it! If you stick with it over the long term, you'll find that you can miss a day or two, or even a week, and get right back on track. There have been times when I have missed my trips to the gym for a week or more, due to other commitments, but I get right back at it with the first possible opportunity. Surprisingly, I never feel as though I missed a beat. The younger version of me would have said this routine does not suit me and I would have quit. Not anymore! As I have aged, I've grown wiser and more patient with myself. When I fall off my exercise program, I get right back on. After all, I am planning for the long run here. And I want my long run to be healthy and happy and ... long!

Body Mass Index (BMI), simply put, is the comparison of a person's weight to height. It is calculated by multiplying body weight by 703 and then dividing by the square of your height in inches. For example, to calculate the BMI for a 100-pound person standing five feet tall: 100 lbs x 703 = 70,300; find the square root of 60 inches = 3600. 70,300 divided by 3600 = 19.52 BMI.

There are many charts, tables and calculators on-line to reference. The standard measures are as follows: Adults with a BMI over 30 are considered obese; adults with a BMI of between 25 and 30 are considered overweight, adults with a

BMI between 18.5 and 25, are considered normal, and adults with a BMI under 18.5 are considered underweight. Another measure, used for women, is waist circumference, where anything below 35 inches is considered to be within a "heart healthy range."

Today's society is obsessed with numbers. However, on the Raw Live Vegan program do not let your scale determine your success. I assure you that weight loss will be a pleasant side effect, starting in the first week of this program. First, you may feel some discomfort as the toxins are gradually eliminated from your system. But continued healthy eating is quickly followed by a heightened level of wellness evidenced by an uplifted mood, balanced blood sugars, lower cholesterol, increased energy, less bloating, clearer thinking, as well as a higher functioning body and increased libido. When it comes to weight loss, you will surpass all of your goals despite your age. In fact, by following this plan, you lose weight despite of yourself

Raw Food For Optimal Health

"The raw food diet is a properly pH-balanced regimen. It's easy to follow, strengthens your immune system, prevents disease, and helps you achieve your ideal weight. Following this program does not mean you will be eating boring, simple foods without taste or savor. The idea is to choose the best foods from the lists and to prepare them in a less damaging way. This will restore your health to a level you perhaps never knew possible."

Raw Live Vegan has given us the ability to create delicious and nutritious meals, desserts and snacks everybody enjoys. The desserts are decadent and the recipes are easy. Should I start with the delicious chocolate desserts or the all-natural sweetener, "Yacan," that actually restores the GI tract and is tolerated by diabetics? Yes, these items are on the raw food diet; although we must consume a broad spectrum of foods to regain optimal vitality and restore health. I personally guarantee you will be satisfied with the level of fullness at the end of the day. You will also satisfy cravings calling-out for something sweet, salty, spicy, creamy or crunchy. It's all here for you to enjoy!

Organization is key to thriving on this lifestyle plan. The grocery list provided on our website outlines what you will need. You will soon find that your shopping habits have changed. You will buy fresh organic produce more often. You will buy bulk items such as seeds, nuts and ground flax. And you will transition your freezer for storing these latter items, as freezing extends their life.

There is a science behind the benefits of the Live, Raw Food Movement. It all comes down to active live enzymes, nutrients, vitamins and chlorophyll that are found in abundance in live sprouts and raw foods. Enzymes create life. They influence every chemical reaction in our body. Enzymes are like worker bees. Without them vitamins, minerals and hormones are unable to perform their essential tasks. Live enzymes supply us with energy, aid in digestion, purify blood and rid the body of waste. Our bodies cannot absorb vitamins without enzymes. Enzymes help us lose weight, lower cholesterol, break down fats, and age gracefully. They detoxify our body, build muscle from protein, and eliminate carbon dioxide from our lungs. They strengthen our immune system and improve our mental capacity. When we cook foods below 118 degrees Fahrenheit, we keep enzymes alive.

Raw food should never be exposed to heat exceeding 118 degrees Fahrenheit. When we eat cooked foods the body uses the enzymes stored in major organs to aid in digestion, depleting our stores and leaving us prone to cancer, coronary heart disease, diabetes and other chronic diseases. The body does its part in supplying enzymes to saliva, as well as gastric, pancreatic and intestinal juices while it's up to us to replenish our system with live enzymes by eating raw food. Some dieticians suggest that stomach acids destroy any live enzyme eaten. Not so, according to Dr. Edward Howell (born in 1898). In 1946 Howell published *The Status of Food Enzymes in Digestion and Metabolism*. In his research he found that when you eat food, acid secretion is minimal for at least thirty minutes. As food travels down the esophagus, it drops into the top part of the stomach - the cardiac section. Each section of the GI tract has a sphincter that allows food to travel at a set time. In this first chamber the live enzymes help self-digestion the most. He also found that it is important to soak your nuts before consumption, as they have natural enzyme inhibitors, which are nature's way of protecting them from premature germination. The enzyme inhibitors protect the species so it can propagate. Dr. Edward Howell and his wife Evangeline both had the appearance, energy and faculties of those 30 years their junior. Do you think he was onto something?

Most bowel diseases stem from a low water-soluble diet. It is important to eat foods high in fibre, such as fresh raw fruits, vegetables, beans and grains, and to be careful how you prepare them. As I noted earlier, do not heat them over 118 degrees Fahrenheit. Also, drink the recommended 6 to 8 glasses of water a day, as water aids digestion. The cause of bowel-related disease is not always diet related. In fact, sometimes bowel diseases stems from a weakness in the wall of the GI tract – anywhere from the esophagus to the colon, where pockets form in the weakness of the GI lining. Food can become trapped and bacteria form when it sits in the pockets of a weak GI tract. One of the most important tasks to promote optimal GI health is regularity! You know your organs are functioning well when what goes in comes out in a timely fashion! Constipation is not good for anyone at any age.

For optimum health, the pH balance requires a more alkaline state to absorb nutrients and oxygen efficiently, and to expel toxins. A diet high in fibre-rich, alkaline foods includes the daily consumption of all of the foods mentioned above and proper preparation. Fibre-rich foods are complex carbohydrates that break down gradually, resulting in less constipation. Foods high in fibre create less wear and tear on the gastrointestinal tract, as they move through the system more quickly than cooked or processed meats and dairy. Fibre also regulates estrogen, as it adheres to it and moves it quickly through the gastrointestinal tract. We all know that obesity contributes to increased estrogen. Estrogen dominant, progesterone depleted is not a good hormonal state to be in, as it contributes to mood swings, decreases libido, increases bloating, weight gain and headaches, and causes tender breasts. Estrogen dominant, progesterone depleted is most common in women entering peri- menopause, who eat a standard North American Diet.

We tax our health care system with preventable ailments like indigestion, high blood sugar, high cholesterol, high blood pressure, arthritis, constipation, fatigue, poor eyesight, poor memory, mood swings, irritability, allergies, brain fog, Candida, depression, and obesity. These conditions are all self-induced, and a result of our poor nutritional intake. Poor nutrition ruins health and sends people running to doctors for a series of prescription medications to treat diseases that, for the most part, could be prevented or even corrected through proper nutrition.

The Fast Food Industry poses the largest threat to our health. The additives (MSG being merely just one of them), high fat and high sugar contents of fast food takes-up (or exceeds) the daily allowable caloric intake all in one sitting. Most fast foods definitely exceed the daily-recommended sugar, salt, and fat contents. And I think we should have a daily limit on additives, that is – if we consume any at all. I'm sure you've read somewhere that nutrients can be *cooked out of* our food. Again, once food is heated beyond 118 degrees Fahrenheit (48 degrees Celsius), the natural enzymes needed to digest foods are killed. Fast cooking at high temperatures – the principle practiced by the fast food industry – changes the amino acid asparagine. This, combined with the sugars in plant foods, results in the formation of acrylamide. Acrylamide causes cancer in laboratory animals. Though tests are not conclusive in humans, more are pending. In light of the research findings for animals, the questions we must ask ourselves are: What is the impact of this chemical on human health? How much of it can we safely consume? How much does it take before it poses a danger on human health? And why doesn't our government move a little faster on banning this type of food preparation? We know people consume this fare on a regular basis. And we all know the real cost of good, nutritious food. So when the fast food industry bates us with outrageously low cost 'meals', what does this say about their quality? It scares me to think about it.

Processed food - now that is a paradox! These two little words should never be used together. At what point do we begin to question and demand our rights to *real* food for ourselves and for our loved ones? Recent recalls of contaminated meat, due to listeriosis or other frightening contaminants such as e-coli or salmonella, are a wake-up call for everyone. The gut is the most abused part of our body. With mindless eating of processed foods, smoking, drug use, and excessive alcohol consumption, people expect to be able to consume whatever they want. Further, they expect their organs will detoxify whatever concoction is consumed as it meanders through the system. Our organs have their limits too. My version of fast food is to enter the local supermarket to buy produce. The choices are great - veggies, fruits, raw nuts... I buy an iced tea, find a bench outside, and enjoy every morsel of nature's fast food, knowing that my organs are grateful for not being stressed to the max.

It is true that we need to eat to live. But, we can reduce the risk of organ damage by eating raw foods. Healthy foods are plentiful and the choices are unlimited. In choosing a Raw Live Vegan lifestyle, we control the quality of food we eat. It is best to choose locally grown, organic fruits and vegetables. Supporting local farmers in their efforts to provide fresh, healthy food is important. Farming co-ops are a "growing trend." I belong to one, where a bin filled with fresh, locally grown produce is dropped off at my front door weekly. The contents vary, so each week there is a new surprise. Through this co-op, I get more fresh produce than I ever did by purchasing retail. I supplement my produce delivery by shopping at local markets for other items that perhaps did not come in my share of crops.

Food grown today is not the same nutritious food grown before fertilizers and chemicals entered the agricultural industry; they were introduced with the hope and promise of higher yields and yes, larger profits for farmers. The phrase 'less is more' rings true when it comes to organics. No, organically farmed foods are not going to be as colourful or as large or as uniform in size and shape as mass-produced foods farmed with the use of chemical sprays and fertilizers that enhance consumer appeal. Fewer chemicals equates to safer, more nutritious food; so less really is more. The environmentally conscious farmer who takes the time to manage crops without the use of chemicals and pesticides deserves our loyal patronage.

I buy local when I can. When I can't, this means I have to trust my local grocer to supply me with organic produce from afar. To buy local and in-season is admirable. But sometimes we have to come to terms with our growing zone, dictated by our climate. In my area, Nova Scotia, the season is short and I must be content with imported produce for several months a year. Again, when I can buy local and in-season, I do. I also enjoy organic fruits and vegetables from afar, such as avocados, mangos, dates and other natural sweeteners. I love food, and I need to be realistic and appreciative of the fact that, by putting the world on my table, I create more appetizing and nutritious recipes. Every day I am grateful for the variety of dishes this abundance provides. Also, it's nice to know I am supporting organic Fair Trade producers in the developing world. I love to purchase their teas and produce. We can't get them here, yet they add unlimited potential to the continuing creativity of my Raw Live Vegan lifestyle.

To fully engage the Raw Food concept of eating you will have to become accustomed to sprouting, dehydrating, and soaking nuts and seeds so they can be safely ingested for optimum nutrition. Sprouting can be a child- friendly task, giving the child the opportunity to learn what real food is and how it arrives from seed or bean to edible protein.

On this site, you will become comfortable with the various concepts of our program in our videos. Browse the resources listed on our website for more in-depth information on raw food and our program. These are resources I used over the past couple of years to enrich my knowledge on this subject. Our resource list will grow over time, as food science is an ongoing study and an ever-evolving journey of discovery for those who continue to be amazed by it. This topic is my personal favourite in reading materials. This lifestyle is not a new trend. In fact, it has been around for a very long time. Published articles on the subject first appeared in the 1920s and 1930s. Momentum continues to build, in light of the current state of our unhealthy population – now desperately turning to this clean way of eating to correct the self-induced damage as a result of mindless eating. I applaud you as you embark on your journey to wellness.

I have nothing but the greatest respect for Bio-Health Diagnostics and the Mayo Clinic and I encourage all to refer to their wealth of knowledge to help when forming decisions on directive of care. My family has benefitted directly from their advisement; my son Bryan's health was restored at a rapid pace, surpassing all expectations in the generalized medical field.

> "By providing people with a glimpse of how you are implementing these powerful choices in your lives, you give healing to many who would otherwise not get it. Your courage, tenacity, diligence, creativity and practical implementation will continue to give you both robust, durable healthy well-being. That is inspirational to me and to anyone interested in healthy well-being."
>
> ~ Dr. J. William LaValley

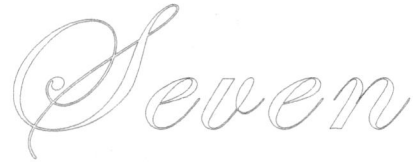

Habits Worth Forming

Journaling for Success

A journal is an important instrument for health and well-being. If well-organized, it can save you and your doctor valuable time. Daily logging of your dietary intake, exercise regimen and feelings gives your doctor the information needed to management your care and to help you establish and pursue long-term health goals without the need for repeat office visits. A journal can be anything from an expensive, hard-covered book with empty lined pages, to a scribbler or a binder filled with loose-leaf notebook paper. If you are serious about finding the answers to your health concerns and making changes to achieve your long-term goals, you will keep a daily journal.

DATE: I start with the middle upper line of each page and write in the day, month and year. In the outer corner of that page, I note the day of my menstrual cycle that I am on. For example, Day 1 might occur on April 5th. It may be Day 1 again on April 30th. For females tracking their cycle, it will show whether you have a full 28-day cycle. Few females do, and this is important information nonetheless. If you happen to go a couple of months without a period it is important to have a record. In this case, your cycle would read something like Day 67, and then Day 1. I also write one-word descriptions of my cycle, for example: heavy or light or trace or cramps, etc. If you no longer have a menstrual cycle, you will obviously omit this step. Your hormone levels are very important to your overall health whether you have a menstrual cycle or not.

NUTRITION: Write down what you eat and when you eat it. This will be unique to your lifestyle and schedule. Not everyone dines at exactly 8:00 a.m., 12-noon and 5:00 p.m. This is desirable, but not always achievable, due to schedules, shift work or demands on time. So write down what you ate and the time of day you actually ate it. Also note whether you were interrupted, and whether you actually got to eat the whole meal or snack. If not, then record how you felt at the time. Were you angry, hungry, frustrated, or indifferent? Is there a pattern – at work or at home – that needs to be addressed? Is there something you can do to better prepare yourself for success? Perhaps with planning you can have readily available finger foods that can be enjoyed. Ideally, this should not be at your desk, but it is better than going without. If interruptions happen at home, then perhaps you have some ideas on shaking-up the routine that no longer works for you.

ACTIVITY: This is a very important section. Regardless of how much, how little, or how often you exercise – write it down. If you have nothing to report, then note any obstacles that got in your way, such as time or energy. It is important to write down something about your level of activity, rather than leaving this section empty. How else will you be able to address this problem? If you write "too tired," this will be valuable information for your doctor. If you write "worked late again," then you have to think of ways to make exercise a priority. Perhaps exercising early in the morning is a solution, or maybe taking time at lunch. If your lunch hour works best, you could eat half of your lunch during your morning break, and the other half in the afternoon. The solution to a busy schedule is easier than you may think. Take the stairs, or walk or bike to and from work. Alternatively, you could park several blocks from the office and walk the rest of the way. If you find that you get too sweaty, then re-think your work wardrobe and wear something that will accommodate this. Any of these options will result in a fitter you, and it will not interfere with valuable family time.

PERSONAL FEELINGS: This section is just as critical as any of the others. Feelings are directly related to nutrition, physical activity and hormones, so writing them down is important. If you are angry – in fact, so angry that you want to duct-tape your mouth to keep from saying something you will regret to some poor innocent soul crossing your path – then write it down. If you are so hungry that you could eat the hind-end off a horse while it's still standing, then write these feelings down too. If you are so tired that you can barely get out of your own way and can't wait for days' end and to curl-up in your pajamas, zoned-out in front of the television (or something equally mindless), then write that down. If you are energized and find yourself preparing supper (in advance) while you finish a workout and mentally multi-task the rest of the week, all at the same time, then write this down too. You do get bragging rights, you know! Never leave this section empty. If you are bored with it all, write it down. This is your time to be honest. When booking your appointment with your family doctor, make it clear that you require adequate time to review your journal, in the hopes of shedding light on your current symptoms.

There is nothing worth discussing with your doctor if you do not have a detailed journal answering the questions asked during a health history of your health complaints. If you don't provide a clear picture of your diet and lifestyle, don't blame your doctor if he is unable to draw conclusions about your health issues. Chances are that he will simply ask you to start a journal and make another appointment.

The Importance of Sleep

Now I lay me down to sleep... How much is enough sleep? Knowing that the recommendation is 7 to 9 hours of sleep each night, and that most people average 6.5 hours, it goes without saying that the majority of us are sleep deprived. Going to bed at 11:00 p.m. and getting up at 6:00 a.m. does not add up to 8 hours of sound sleep. It takes most people half an hour, on average, to prepare for bed. It takes another 30 to 45 minutes to unwind, especially if you have a partner. So if you're planning on 8 hours of sleep, you need to consider the extra time it takes to settle in.

Have you ever heard the term 'sleeping like a baby?' A baby enjoys 50% of their sleep in what is called Rapid Eye Movement (REM) sleep. This is where the limbs don't move, but the eyelids do. REM is a form of deep sleep. Adults only enjoy 20% of sleep in this state.

If you're having trouble sleeping, consult your doctor. Before you go, keep a journal of what you eat, how much you sleep, how much activity you get, and how much you work outside of the house, and take it to your appointment. Your doctor is your confidant. Share with him or her your feelings, good or bad. If you are feeling tired, but still don't sleep well, have your blood work checked.

You might be suffering from low iron or a thyroid condition. Lack of sleep can cause serious health issues, such as foggy thinking, impaired memory, depression, and suppressed immunity. Lack of sleep also exacerbates chronic pain, particularly when the pain isn't being treated.

If you are one of the majority who averages 6.5 hours of sleep a night, then plan to nap some time during the day to make up for this deficit. This should be a priority, until you have reached the recommended 7 to 9 hours of sleep each night.

Stress plays a huge role in sleep deprivation. Ignoring our stressors will not make them go away. Rather, face them straight on. Think about the issues that are stressing you and write them down. Then think about and list the steps you can take to alleviate them. If there is more than one stressor, write them down in their order of magnitude. Try to figure out which stressor impacts you the most and which one is the most benign. Be sure to leave room beside each stressor, on your list, to write an action plan.

Stress affects each of us in different ways. One person's stress could be another person's cakewalk, depending on our individual natures and situations. Stress is also what you believe it to be. Knowing your stressors, and having a plan in mind to deal with them, is half the battle. Anticipating a stressful situation and knowing, ahead of time, how you are going to deal with it will reduce your anxiety and help you sleep.

Your bedroom should be set up for sleep. Ask yourself whether it is conducive to sleep or whether it is set up as a multi- media entertainment centre. Do you have a computer that sits on a desk in your bedroom? Does it entice you to check those late night e-mails or to log into *Facebook* for a late night chat with a 'friend?' No matter how tired you are, tapping away on your computer, and reading on line posts or messages, sends your mind into wake up mode. Computers have no down time; they don't need to sleep. So train yourself to shut yours down and log in the next day. All of those messages and posts can wait. You might also consider locating your computer somewhere else. Computers are nasty; they go into different modes during the night, and they emit heat and light. You may think that your computer is not disturbing your sleep, but it is. It pulls you from that deep REM sleep, where your body re-energizes and boosts your immunities, to a shallow stage of sleep, somewhere between REM and wakefulness.

Having a television in your bedroom can be just as bad. If you think that you can drift off in front of a late night show, you are only fooling yourself. Even if you do drift off, at some point, the background noise will nudge you awake and remind you to get up and turn the television off. Finally, that iron, ironing board and basket of wrinkled laundry have to go. There is nothing worse on the psyche than a tedious chore that beckons you from the corner of your bedroom.

Exercise is good for you, but if you are not sleeping well, then you need to assess when you are fitting it into your schedule. Exercising late at night energizes you and keeps you awake long after you have finished your session. If you have a busy work life, it is best to exercise early in the morning. You may feel like you're sleepwalking to the gym, after that early morning alarm. But once you have completed your routine and hit the shower, you will experience that feeling of euphoria and clear headedness that helps you organize your day and take on anything that it throws at you. Also, exercising early in the morning leaves you guilt free, as it does not cut into precious family time, an important consideration for those of us who work. Learn to prioritize and put yourself first. At the end of the day, you will have time for friends and family. It's not too often that they want your attention at 5:00

a.m. To make it easier to get to that early morning exercise session, on a consistent basis, consider pairing up with someone who has the same goals as you do and whom you can depend on to be there consistently.

Statistics have proven that people who exercise regularly have better coping skills than those who don't. Exercise pumps oxygen to all parts of the body, propelling it toward peak performance, depending on the intensity and duration of the exercise. Your skin will radiate with that special glow that comes from a healthy lifestyle.

If you're worried about getting to work on time, pack your work clothes in a carry on bag so they won't wrinkle. And do yourself a favor and adopt a no fuss hair do; this cuts down on half the battle. If you car pool, then take advantage of lunch time to get outside for the natural light that boosts serotonin. The more natural light you get each day, the better you will sleep at night.

Nutrition plays a huge role in sleep. Caffeinated coffee should not be consumed at night, as it will keep you awake; a nice herb tea is a better option. Avoid high fat, high carbohydrate, processed foods at night; your body will spend half the night digesting them. Some people believe a good stiff alcoholic drink will put them into sleep mode. This is true, but only until it metabolizes, then it wakes you up.

Adopting a relaxing routine at the end of your day will help you sleep. I start winding down as early as possible, preferably at 8:00 p.m. Yes, I'm lucky to be an empty nester. But I take pride in this time; it is leisurely and I feel pampered, as it is just for me. I set my alarm and double check it (I'm a little obsessive-compulsive disordered when it comes to time). I keep my alarm clock in my bathroom for two reasons; first, I don't like the light that the digital clock shines into my room. Second, I don't want to keep checking it to see if the power has gone off or whether it's time to get up. As my bathroom is an *ensuite*, I can hear the alarm clock from there. After I set my alarm, I take a nice, warm Epsom salts bath. Sometimes I pamper myself with a facemask, or a foot scrub. Then I soak for a while, and read a good book until the water cools. If the book is really good, I add hot water and soak some more. Then I slip into my nice, roomy, cotton pajamas, (I know, too much information!). I like to meditate before crawling into bed. I do a little deep breathing, to quiet myself down, and I think about all of the things that I am grateful for. This sends me into a nice, deep, peaceful sleep. Good Night, Sleep Tight!

Stress Reducing Strategies

Stress is a part of everyday life, as it's all around us. There are good stressors and bad stressors. The key is to differentiate between the two and reduce the bad ones.

Good stressors are necessary for everyday life. They are the ones that get you to work on time, put food on the table, pay the bills, attend to household chores, and organize ourselves and our families. Sometimes change can bring on stress, even when it is a good stress. A new job, a move or a new relationship can cause good stress. Sometimes this change is something we unwittingly initiate, such as becoming so proficient in our job that we are offered a raise and or a promotion. The stress comes in facing longer work hours, being assigned more responsibility or having to move to another city, and wondering what the impact will be on our family. A lesser positive stressor could occur after we have developed a healthy routine of physical exercise or an interesting hobby, and a like minded-person asks to join. This compels us to decide whether we need to rearrange our schedule, or make room for someone else in an activity we might prefer to do alone. These are low level stressors, but stressors nonetheless, as they require change. But change is inevitable. In life, nothing stays the same; people come and go; new businesses are established, others fold; whole communities can be established, others die. Consider the constant change our forefathers faced as pioneers, some of it good, but much of it highly stressful. We are the direct descendants of these early survivors, which means that we are conditioned to take on whatever stress life throws our way.

Bad stressors can stem from incidents beyond our control, like the loss of a loved one. This is an unfortunate situation that often requires professional help, particularly when the death is of a spouse or a child; or if it is sudden or violent. These latter stressors may require coping mechanisms in therapy and in prescription drugs. Eventually, time heals the worst wounds, but in the interim professional help is often necessary and highly recommended. It is best to be open, so that you can get help from someone you trust.

When using medication to relieve stress, it is important to follow the guidelines set out by your doctor. Read about the drug, so that you know what the side effects are. If you have a negative reaction to it, see your doctor right away. He or she will prescribe another medication developed for the same purpose that may not affect you adversely. Never stop a medication cold turkey, as this can result in negative side affects. If you have thoughts of discontinuing a drug, do so with the help of your doctor.

Bad stressors can also occur when we allow things to spiral out of control. Typically these stressors are our own doing. They might include committing ourselves to something we don't have time for or know little about, or purchasing something that throws a wrench into the household budget.

Keeping up with the Jones's is one of today's classic stressors. Allowing someone else to influence our wants and needs can send us into a downward spiral of personal financial destruction. If you allow 'The Jones's' to influence your purchases, you will soon find yourself in the same dark financial abyss as these seemingly wealthy people. Purchasing things spontaneously on credit offers a fleeting moment of happiness. But the pain of facing credit card debt at the end of each month lasts much longer. It also sends a message of false security to the rest of the family, where they come to believe that there is no end to what they can have. Often we find that we cannot pay off the monthly balance. The bad stressor kicks in when we find that our credit card debt has accumulated so much, and that the interest charges on the balance are so high, that important and necessary purchases must be put aside because the money has already been spent. The more difficult this becomes, the greater the stress. At some point the consequences of frivolous spending can affect family and spousal relationships.

There are times when an unnecessary purchase becomes a must. The fair way to deal with the issue would be to gather everyone around the kitchen or dining room table for a discussion. If the item is important enough, something must be given up, such as cable TV. Some may be willing to sell off items that may be in good condition, yet have piled up in the garage or basement unused. You could gather them up, have a yard sale, make some money and get a clean basement or garage in the process! This method ends up becoming a valuable lesson in household finance, and a skill your children will adopt, as they grow and mature and face life's challenges.

Overdue Accounts, stress enhancer, are easy to tackle if you design a system that allows you to budget according to your payday. Perhaps you may opt to pay bills on line or set up a direct withdrawal at your bank. Keep an eye on your budget, and set priorities. If, for example, your cosmetic budget is getting out of hand, shop around for less expensive services. Or, you could do your own manicure or hair coloring. Have a spa day with the family. Invite friends over and have some fun! Other ways to reduce stress are to take your own lunch to work, and to prepare your children's lunch at home, rather than resorting to the workplace or school cafeteria. These options are less expensive and they

are far healthier. Prepare lunches the night before. And while you're at it, you could lay out your clothes and plan your breakfast, to avoid that morning crunch. There's nothing worse than waking up to find that the clothes you wanted to wear are dirty, and that there is no coffee in the pantry when you have a household to rally!

Some stressors are easier to handle than others. Take household chores, for example. This kind of stress can lend to positive family relationships, as a schedule is set, chores are divvied up, and everyone works together for a common purpose. Be sure to choose a time that works for everyone. Rotate the tasks so that the skill sets are learned by all. There's nothing like a clean house when the chores are finished. Everyone is happier, and then focus turns to food.

Food preparation in the kitchen should include everyone. This is a time when family members can talk about their day, learn a little home economics, and perhaps assert their own creativity, which should always be rewarded. Food preparation teaches your children how to budget. They learn the wisdom of measuring ingredients so there is little waste. They also learn that left over ingredients can go back into the fridge for another meal. This can also be a time to plan ahead, where two meals are whipped up and one is frozen for that future busy day.

If work is the problem, talk to your boss about the possibility of getting some help. Perhaps the job requires an extra set of hands or an upcoming course that will allow you to handle a new responsibility with ease and confidence. Perhaps it could be something as simple as working on a different schedule. If all fails, in trying to make the best of a difficult workplace situation, start looking elsewhere. Be sure to ask for a copy of your annual appraisal, so that you can use it as a current reference.

You owe it to yourself to sit down and create your own stress lists, good and bad, and to write down what you're going to do to ease them. Encourage your loved ones to do same, regardless of how young they are. For example, the child with the responsibility of taking the puppy out to void, could leave their outdoor wear and a collar and lead conveniently by the back door. Providing logical and convenient spaces for important items that are used communally is a huge stress reducer, particularly when everyone honors the system.

We as people fall into automatic pilot mode with life in general, nose to the grind stone, go to work, clean house, shop, prepare meals etc., etc., etc. But there comes a time when we ponder our new stations in life that we can implement change! Perhaps for some it is the stage of empty nest. You will notice a difference in your grocery bill for one. This is a time where you may re-evaluate many things. Perhaps you are living in a house that is larger than what you need and downsizing may be the thing to do. Perhaps you may now want to move from the suburbs to the inner city to be close to all things and not require the car so much when everything is in walking distance! You at this very special time in your life can go from "it's all about the kids" to "it's all about me!" Now there's a thought!

Stress has a different meaning for everyone. When my daughter was younger, she used to say to me, when I was feeling stressed, "Take a chill pill Mom!" Now that she has become a mature young woman, she says, "Breathe Mom, breathe from your abdomen, deep in and then let it go!" How simple, yet how effective!

Travelling Healthfully

Regardless of how much or how little we travel we should automatically consider health promoting planning in our packing, indeed a necessary habit! Travel permits us to check out the hidden wonders of the world's culinary delights. It is nice to pack something to take along, but better to open ourselves up to local cuisine. Traveling healthfully can be done. As food sustains and energizes us, we need it for basic survival. The wrong food leaves us feeling depleted, bloated, constipated and generally unwell. So plan first and foremost around food, and be in charge of the outcome. Planning ahead means becoming familiar with health food stores, supermarkets, and vegan and Asian restaurants in the region we are visiting. Most regions offer a wide range of fresh fruits and vegetables. Finding these sources helps us stay on course during our holiday. Most of these sources can be found on the Internet. With planning WE are in charge of the outcome.

Historically, vacations have been a time to break from the mundane responsibilities of job and home. We give ourselves permission to relax, to gorge on local food and to imbibe local drink. We leave our regular duties behind us, which frees us to partake in healthy pursuits without interference. We can spend the whole day in our active wear if we want to. But, as carefree as a vacation may be, we still need to think about food.

We think nothing of packing a curling iron and hairdryer, so why not pack a handheld blender too? This handy, compact kitchen tool will help prepare our morning shake and afternoon wheatgrass juice in minutes. If we want to enjoy a happy, healthy vacation and return feeling rested and refreshed, we must pack for success. If we do not plan, we plan to fail.

On cruises, family visits, and short local trips we are all at the mercy of hotels and local dining rooms. Make sure the room has a kitchenette. Be bold and ask room service to leave fruit on the pillow instead of chocolates. Check the local directory for vegan choices and check out menus before committing. Asian restaurants are an excellent choice.

Ask them to fill their seaweed wraps with vegetables only. Frequent the local markets and health food stores, and pick up delicious, fresh, organic fruits and vegetables to take back to the room. Many grocery stores stock fresh sprouts, herbs, salad greens, and the best of fruits and green teas. What more could we ask for.

Staying active while on vacation is important too. Check out local activities and gyms. There are often bike trails, bike rentals and seasonal rentals such as skates, skis, kayaks or canoes. Take a camera and a map, and make the trip one to remember. If we put these simple plans in place and our vacation will surely be a success.

The following is a list of suggested items for travel:
- *Greens Plus* for morning shake.
- Zip-lock bag of mixed cereal groats to soak.

- Mung beans to sprout, where there is fresh water, one can sprout in a wide mouth thermos, leave lid loose.
- Concentrated wheat grass powder, for mid-afternoon pick me up.
- Hormone supplements.
- "L'A'RABAR" this is an energy bar with minimal ingredients and no chemicals. This is a guilt-free indulgence that is great for on the airplane or if you are stuck somewhere. It will hold you over.
- Pedometer, sneakers, sunglasses and stainless steel thermos.

Beware of Burnout

Burnout is a state of perpetual exhaustion that stays with us all day even after a good night's sleep. Over time, burnout affects our health, as it plays on our immune system and leaves us prone to colds and flu. It is important to recognize burnout for what it is, because it affects you and those around you, both at work and at home, in many ways.

Feelings of burnout creep up on you unawares. You might sense a dark cloud hovering over you, and feel that you can't shake the doom and gloom it brings. Maybe you feel invisible, you think that nobody recognizes the good you do, and you wonder why you bothered doing it in the first place. Or you think that what you're doing is meaningless and you're just too tired to care. Or maybe you're past that point. Maybe you feel so detached that you have become emotionally uninvolved with situations that would otherwise affect you, such as when a friend or loved one is awarded an important bonus or promotion or loses a job. If you find that your emotions are numbed to major events that impact those around you, if you feel uncharacteristically detached from issues that are important to them, then you are most likely experiencing burnout. If so, now is the time to seek help in addressing this serious issue.

If you believe the problem stems from work, then talk to your supervisor. Burnout is a health issue; there are allowances for time off. Perhaps your workload is severe. Perhaps more has been delegated to you than time permits, and you find yourself working through your breaks in order to complete these new tasks. Maybe your work has become repetitive and tedious, and you no longer find it stimulating. Review your responsibilities with your supervisor, to determine whether they are reasonable. If you feel as if you are stuck in a rut, ask for a new assignment. If this is not possible, look elsewhere, before you crash or worse end up with a bad reference.

Meditation is a time to get in touch with your inner child. It will ease a heavy day, as its wonderful calming effect induces relaxation and inner peace. It can be done anywhere and for whatever amount of time you might have to enjoy it. Or, perhaps there is a hobby, craft or other favorite pastime you no longer pursue. Make the time. Indulging in recreation may just be the thing you need to take your mind off work. Being a 'yes' or a 'go to' person is not necessarily the best person to be. There are times when it is better to fly a tad 'under the radar,' where you do your job and you're not taken to task. We all know people like that. They're the faded grey between the black and white. They're the subtle tone of wallpaper that blends in with the office furniture. They come to work, they do their job, and they collect their paycheck. They don't complain, they never gossip, and no one ever speaks good or ill of them. And they leave the office, every Friday afternoon, just as fresh and energetic as they were on Monday morning. Chances are that they have a more exciting life outside of the office. They're likely saving all that extra energy for fulfillment elsewhere. In any event, their lives are, no doubt, far more well-rounded than ours.

We all have things we need to do to pay the bills, and we are all aware of the things that bring us joy. The healing is in the balance. Even if we're lucky enough to be doing a job that we love, we should be disciplined enough to give so much of ourselves and no more. If we don't, we run the risk of burnout. Most of us work to pay the bills. In today's economy, many of us work long hours just to make ends meet. But, it is important to find the balance between work and enjoyment. To be truly happy, we need to find fulfillment elsewhere; we need to play. At the end of each day think of ways you can reward yourself for a job well done, and then make the time to enjoy them. Also, think of the things you are truly grateful for. In a state of burnout there may not be many, but recognizing one thing would be a good start. Be good to yourself, and strive for balance!

> "I have thought much about the information that you have written and you have done a great job. You have accumulated superb documentation and I'd like to discuss with you and Phil my comments."
>
> ~ Dr. J. William LaValley

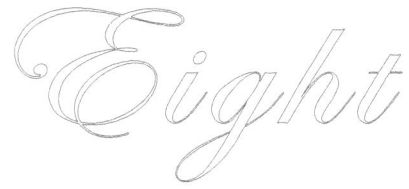

Motivation

Retrain The Brain

Holistically, our brain and body must be in sync, as we embrace this new lifestyle. We need to adjust our way of thinking and eating despite how we were raised, what we have become used to and what the media has taught us. To move forward, into a more positive, healthful direction, we should shed all things negative.

Over the years, my wardrobe has expanded to include lots of exercise clothing, as spending so much time at the gym has become part of the enjoyment of my new, healthy lifestyle. It's especially nice to have a couple of changes ready to go. Presents on my wish list have changed from jewelry, to gym memberships, gift certificates at sports shops, home equipment, such as yoga DVDs, yoga mats, good running shoes and a bike for outdoor excursions. When Phil and I travel, our footwear has changed from heels and dress shoes, to hiking shoes. Our jackets are now multi-layered, and multi-functional, to meet the change of climate and weather conditions in distant locales.

You have one life to live, and it is your choice to live it well, so don't waste time. As the Nike commercial says - Just do it! Enlightenment is for anyone who searches truth on his or her jour- 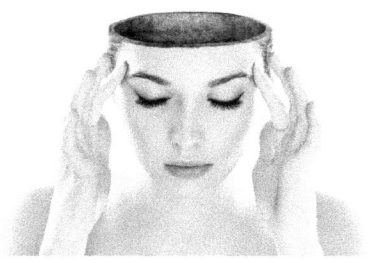 ney through life. With each new concept you introduce into your current lifestyle, you will gain momentum to continue introducing more. Fearlessly and tirelessly, you will evolve into exactly what it is that you perceive yourself to be. Think of someone who is truly healthy and envision what his or her pantry would contain. Now think about how they would plan out their week, in their day-timer. Do you think they would set aside time for exercise, meal preparation, and time for them to reflect on a week well done? You bet they would, and so should you!

As you move down in size, donate your clothes to a charity. After all, this is a permanent shift in your lifestyle, and you won't need those oversized clothes anymore. The change will not happen overnight, but it will gradually become evident that this new you is here to stay. What is the current literature lining your shelves and coffee tables? Does it speak about the new you? If not, get rid of it. Read something new in the line of self-empowerment. You can learn a lot from this kind of literature, as it often sheds light on why we are the way we are, and includes great tips on moving beyond it. It also offers suggestions as to how to stay on track without offending friends and family. They will simply have to get used to the new you.

When I grocery shop, I take my time. I use a list, but I also keep an open mind for the wonderful surprises I might find as I scan the isles. I am always excited when something new arrives. Perhaps 'new to me' excites my adventurous side. I then plan a meal that incorporates this new item. There's nothing like taking the ho-hum out of grocery shopping. I put this new item into my cart, as a point of pride, knowing that I will be using the best products to serve to my family and friends.

Deep down, we humans are independent in thought and deed. Despite being united in societal, familial and individual relationships, we all have control over our own destiny. We are free to make connections with new circles that grow our friendships. The circles of friends we choose says a lot about who we are, so we must choose them well. To break out of conformity is not only healthy, it is inspiring. It is a feeling of self- control, enthusiasm, passion and purpose. Use your purpose and new knowledge to move in a direction that is self- sustaining, and give yourself a big hug.

Self Image

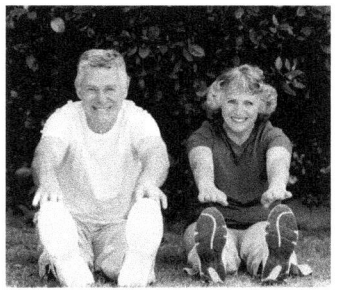

Self Image is the mental picture we have of ourselves. It is also how we perceive others see us. Self image is very interesting. Starting from childhood, imposed by self and by others, our self image is often resistant to change. Some questions you might ask, in relation to your own self-image are: Is your self-image skewed? When looking into the mirror, do you see fat when others see a fit lean body? Or is your self-image based on a strong, nurturing environment, where you were encouraged to develop skills and to recognize your strengths? This latter environment is one that helps mould us into strong, confident, sociable and independent people, prepared to make a positive contribution to society.

Poor self-image is brought on by a lifetime of negative criticisms from friends, from family and from acquaintances. As adults, we know that a person's propensity to criticize says more about their need to do so, than it says about us. But, as children lack this level of reasoning and self-awareness, they often take criticisms, from an adult, as truths; thus the damage caused.

Humans are societal beings. We interact with others, on a daily basis, and we depend on each other. The idea behind our personal development is that it should prepare us to interact effectively within society; this means cooperating with and supporting each other in the home, in social settings and in the work force. Most people we have daily contact with are not privy to how our background has shaped us. We tend to guard our more intimate information and only share it at a more personal level. If rejection happens, then we guard our innermost secrets even more.

Victimization has a detrimental impact on self-image. Self-image deteriorates, precipitously, under the strain of abuse or when in a situation of manipulation that leaves us feeling helpless and pessimistic. Feelings of guilt or self-blame also come into play. All of these images and feelings are shaped by how we are treated by others. When victimization leads to despair, which it generally does, professional help is encouraged. The problem is that we often don't see ourselves as being victimized at the outset, as we are too trusting. It is only when we are well into a bad situation, when we recognize our plight. Sadly, by that time, we are so beaten down that we often have little energy to fight back or to seek help. Access to information on victimization is a problem for many, as they do not know which way to turn. If we see someone being victimized, it is our duty to offer support and guidance. Ultimately, we are interconnected. Society cannot function adequately if we don't recognize the important roll we each play in it. We are individuals and also a society. We are the trees and also the forest. Unfortunately, some of us don't see it that way.

When looking in the mirror silence the messages and the thoughts of perception imposed by self or others. Still yourself and just be, accepting who are, you ARE you, love yourself.

Six Degrees of Wellness

"How many times have you seen someone whom you believe to be healthy, based on appearance, only to find that their poor health was masked by a thin body, make-up and great clothes? And how many times have you tried to attain this same 'look' of optimal health through sacrifice, denial and following the latest diet trend promoted in yet another #1 national best seller, when you know that what you are really presenting is a false image?"

Our outward appearance is what people see first. It is often how they read us and judge us. Appearances can lead us (and others) to believe we are really healthy, when in fact we could be masking or avoiding a serious health issue. Coming from a nursing background, I know that external appearance doesn't always tell the true story of a person's state of health. It's our inner health that really counts. It's the knowledge we gain, in our quest for optimal health, and the choices we make, on this journey that determine how healthy we really are. But to know where we really are, health-wise, it all boils down to blood work.

A healthy body starts with good nutrition, hormonal balance and an active lifestyle.

Nutritionally, it is best to go organic, so that your body is exposed to as few toxins as possible. Eliminate sugar, eat as much raw food as possible, and make sure that your digestive supplements include enzymes that will keep your GI tract healthy. Hormonal panels should also be done. These are scheduled blood tests taken over a specified period of time to determine hormone levels. Women should start having their hormonal panels done in their thirties or earlier if medically required. Men should start them in their forties. This requires regular blood work, which provides a comparison of hormonal ranges as they change over time. This information will allow your doctor to recommend necessary adjustments, be they dietary or through bio-identical hormone therapy.

Blood work tells the real truth about your health. It provides your doctor with a window into what is going on inside of your body, and helps him to determine a course of action that will help you regain your health. Blood work is used to measure active and inactive hormone levels, blood sugar and cholesterol levels. It detects allergies, pathogens and some cancers. It also tests for heart attack and for liver and kidney function. Regular blood work helps your doctor track your progress and determine whether adjustments in therapies or supplements are needed. It is an important factor in the quest for optimal health.

Regular exercise also enhances health and wellbeing. It decreases risk of disease, as it boosts immunities. It increases energy, and improves stamina, self-esteem, mental health, and focus. It also increases metabolism, improves muscle tone and body shape, and adds radiance to our complexion.

Motivation

Good nutrition, hormonal balance and regular exercise work together to determine our current level of wellness.

Levels of wellness range from 'high', at one end of the health spectrum, to 'death' on the other end. Most of us are neither totally healthy nor totally ill at any given time. And most of us fall within ranges that are considered acceptable, for our age group and gender, by current medical standards. The problem is that current medical standards are not measures of optimal health. They are ranges of measures that have been adjusted, over time, to accord with changes in our western lifestyle. And you know that some of these changes have included unhealthy convenience foods and a less physical activity that accommodate increasingly busy schedules.

Your family doctor could tell you that your level of wellness is perfectly acceptable, and that you have nothing to worry about, when the state of your health is actually far from optimal. My husband and I have been in that situation. We have been told that we fit within acceptable ranges, health-wise, when we really felt unwell. I'm sure that many of you have had the same experience. It's time to wake up and face the reality of reduced standards in health measurements, and take your personal well being into your own hands. If you have faced a serious health issue, some time in your life, and have been willing to have it managed strictly through pharmaceuticals, without making a personal effort to correct the cause of your illness, then this program is not for you. But, if you are not accepting of our current, pharmaceutically driven health care system, if you want to take control of your own health, and if you are willing to do this through optimal nutrition and hormonal balance, with natural therapy (if required), then this program is for you.

We all have experienced illness. Some of us have might even have been near death's door. But it is the desire to attain

High Level Wellness that separates us from the majority. Fuelling your body with optimal nutrition will help you achieve this goal. Once you know what it is that is making you sick, then it is up to you to make the necessary changes that will help you regain your health. I would never suggest going off a prescribed medication; that is dangerous. My objective is to help you improve your health naturally, so that your doctor can reduce your need for medication, gradually and healthfully. I want to help you develop the tools that will permit you to take ownership of your own health, and decide where you want to be in the **Six Degrees of Wellness.**

Levels of Wellness
High Level Wellness
Good Health
Normal Health
Illness
Critical Health
Death

High Level Wellness starts with good physical self-care. You can achieve High Level Wellness if you adopt the necessary components to do this. You could start by listing the things that you do that are good for your health. (Reading this article and contemplating this program is a good start.) Next, consider what constitutes good physical self-care. Are you eating nutritiously? Are organic products first on your grocery list? Do you avoid harmful chemicals? Do you know which chemicals are harmful and in which products they are found? Are you dependent on a prescription drug? Do you get enough sleep? The first signs of aging

are lack of muscle tone. With this in mind, do you make exercise enough and is it a priority? Are you working and playing safely? Prevention of illness and injury should be a priority. Do you get regular checkups according to your age and gender? Are you aware of any family health history that points to potential problems now or in the near future?

Your mental health is important too. It's important to be intellectually stimulated and it's important to be happy. Do you make time, during the day, to spend with loved ones and do things that you enjoy? Keeping yourself engaged in stimulating activities and having positive interaction with others is good for strong mental health.

When thinking about the state of your mental health, you could start by asking yourself what your interests are. Are they nutrition, wellness, the environment, the arts, or craft-related? Ask yourself if you using your full intellectual potential. If not, find an interesting hobby and delve into it. No matter what your interests are, the brain needs to be exercised.

Everyday we are bombarded with mixed messages that tell us that 'You only live once, so enjoy yourself !' or 'Life is so short, live a little, the gym will be there waiting for you tomorrow!' or 'This one meal won't hurt you!' Remember the fable about the ant and the cricket? The ant spent months gathering and storing grain for the long winter. The cricket chose to sing all summer long. The cricket's laziness caused him to be unprepared when winter came. But this is a choice he made. The fable tells us that, as the cricket didn't take responsibility for his long-term needs, he met with a very sad end. The moral of this fable is that we suffer the consequences of the choices we make. We can use this same lesson for ourselves when we are making lifestyle choices that affect our health. Ultimately, we are all responsible for our own personal choices. When we come into contact with something unhealthy, we can either partake of it or we can abstain. The decisions we make, inevitably determine our

Level of Wellness. Only you can make the changes that enhance your own personal health.

It's the little things you do each day that make the biggest changes. Requesting that a particular item be stocked at your local grocery store is one small step in the right direction. Being aware of safety at work is another step. For example, if you notice that something is being handled unsafely at work, you need to speak out. This action could prevent you or someone else from being needlessly injured. The gift of knowledge comes the responsibility to do the right thing for yourself and also for those around you.

Using reliable knowledge around you, such as getting a second opinion on a health matter, is also important. Sometimes it can be life altering. I have witnessed people suffering from a serious health issue, rise to a High Level of Wellness, because they invested time and energy into investigating a problem that their family doctor couldn't adequately address. They embraced their newfound knowledge in issues of wellness and achieved success.

Emotional health is also important. Emotional pain and stress in our everyday lives are unique to each one of us. They can sometimes be so huge that we feel as if we carry the weight of the world on our shoulders. The ability to think things through, and to write down what our situation is, how we got there and how it is affecting us is very important. It's also important not to burden those around us with our emotional problems. This is where expressing emotions on how you feel at the right time and the right place is important. Talking with a trained healthcare professional who has the ability to assess your emotional health is best the way to effect change. Complaining to those around you is ineffective. You place an undue burden on family and friends when you do this, and it won't help you with your situation.

Motivation

Comfortable and congenial interpersonal relationships are important to personal wellness. We are never alone when we have friends. Human touch is important to emotional health. But mental stress that causes anger doesn't permit this. It is important to recognize the source of your anger and to deal with it appropriately, instead of projecting your anger on innocent people around you. How you engage yourself in your day often dictates its outcome. If you wake up bitter and angry, and project this onto those around you, you may push them away. If this condition persists and you don't seek professional help, you may find that you compromise the very relationships that are important for your own emotional health.

Health and lifestyle choices today are intrinsically linked to the environment and the broader world around us. When considering our lifestyle choices, whether it be about food, energy, or material consumption, we need to think about whether they are sustainable. We have to set our own pace, when making health and lifestyle choices, but we can also be instruments of change, through the choices we make. We can make choices that benefit the environment and ourselves. And as we gain new knowledge, and change one bad habit at a time, we can share it with others. With each new change we will build momentum, move rapidly up the Levels of Wellness, achieve optimal health, and create a healthier world in the process.

Most of us move up and down the Six Levels of Wellness during life's journey. Obtaining the knowledge to set you onto a pathway to good health is an excellent start. Once you are on this road, you will find that there is so much that you have control over. And in the event that bad health comes your way, you will be in the best condition, both mentally and physically, to take on this new challenge in a positive way.

The more prepared you are, the better the outcome with be. Starting with a positive disposition and a healthy dose of knowledge has its advantages as you move up The Six Degrees of Wellness.

This Subject of Aging

We are living in a time when great strides are being made on the subject of aging. It has become a hot topic, especially among baby boomers, as they present a huge and lucrative market. Lifestyle products and services have been heavily focused on this particular group. And as boomers are individuals with a broad range of tastes and needs, the options presented to them are countless.

There are three schools of thought on aging. For some, aging well means taking life as it comes and accepting it, regardless of how difficult it can be. For others, it means being proactive and taking steps to prevent age- related health issues before they arise. These people make a huge effort to maintain a good quality of life. Still others, when they reach life's autumn, want to turn back the clock and enjoy more youthful vigor. They are the adventurous types who are willing to embrace a new lifestyle, regardless of how radically different it can be.

For those who wish to take life as it comes and maintain a lifestyle replete with a poor diet and addictive vices that play on their health, particularly as they age, there is the pharmacy. Pharmaceuticals alone can manage a variety of diseases and prolong life. This does not mean, for a second, that people in this camp do not enjoy a good life. Some of them do, but they are few. Perhaps their happy-go-lucky personality allows them to defeat the odds. Or it could be a great set of genes. But statistics tell us that the majority of those

Motivation

who drink, smoke and eat bad food meet an early grave. And those who do manage to survive into old age live with a variety of ailments that severely limit their quality of life.

The second group of aging boomers is the one that chooses a preventative lifestyle. These people read widely and anticipate the aches, pains and inconveniences that come with aging. They exercise, they limit their vices, and they follow good nutrition. Some wish to avoid the pitfalls of inherited genes. Others simply wish to stay healthy and age as gracefully and painlessly as possible.

The third group is the one that I will call 'the young at heart.' They are curious, intelligent and adventurous. Some would call them Mavericks, as they want to try cutting edge techniques and turn back the clock. I would put myself, and anyone following the Raw Live Vegan program, into this group. But regardless of whether you are adventurous or simply proactive, there is something unique, yet simple and affordable, that we can all do in our fight against aging: it is to embrace optimal nutrition. Nutrition is vital to optimal aging. It slows the signs of aging and feeds the soul.

Good nutrition should include a variety of raw foods. It should also include supplements because, as we age, we lose the ability to process vitamin B. A deficiency in vitamin B leads to heart disease and memory loss. But before we decide on a supplement regimen it is imperative to have an annual consultation with a physician for blood work. Blood work will show if you are deficient in vitamins and minerals. Your doctor will then design a supplement regimen to add to your diet.

Raw, fresh, organic fruits, vegetables and legumes offer a plethora of anti-oxidants and live enzymes that boost your immunities and help you fight off the free radicals that you come in daily contact with. Anti-oxidants are our first line of defense against free radicals that cause pre-mature aging, health problems and even cancer. Fruits and vegetables also contain natural carbohydrates that keep you energized, water that benefits the skin, and fiber that moves food easily through the GI tract.

Fruits and vegetables are best eaten raw. A raw salad is full of vitamins, nutrients and anti-oxidants, making it one of the healthiest dietary choices and a key to anti-aging. If you are not preparing your own salad, be sure that it is served with simple vinaigrette of olive oil, vinegar and a few spices, served on the side. Ask that any extras, such as forbidden dairy, meat or processed croutons be excluded. Hopefully your salad will come with a healthy serving of tomatoes.

The tomato is a Superfood with anti-aging properties that are off the charts. It is power- packed with vitamin A, also known as retinol, which is known to protect the eyes, skin and brain. Tomatoes also contain vitamin C, beta-carotene, potassium, thiamine, calcium, and the anti-oxidant lycopene. Lycopene promotes healthy organs. It also aids our skin by producing melanin, which protects us from UV damage - a definite aging factor. Potassium helps us maintain water balance and electrolytes. It also helps prevent strokes, maintain blood pressure, reduce anxiety and stress, increase metabolism, and regulate heart and kidney function. Thiamine helps maintain a healthy nervous system and aids cardiovascular function. Calcium is necessary for strong bones and teeth.

The Raw Live Vegan program is rich in vitamins and anti-oxidants. With its hydrating foods, green teas and water, it aids in hydrating our bodies, which is also key to anti-aging. To learn more about the benefits of the variety of foods on this program, read the chapters on 'Superfoods' and 'Vitamins and Minerals.'

Feeling young and living life to its fullest means different things to different people. Many of us look beyond nutrition in the quest to stay young. For some, exercise and good nutrition are enough. In this fast paced society some are continually reinventing themselves, as they seek out the latest treatments that promise to banish all signs of aging. Granted some of these options feed the ego and strip us of our hard earned money. But many aging-related treatments that may seem cosmetic actually benefit our health. One of these is stripping varicose veins. Superficial veins can usually be ignored. But deep veins, if left untreated, can cause blood clots that can result in a life threatening pulmonary embolism. Another corrective treatment is laser surgery to correct eye vision. This is a Godsend for those who do tedious tasks that cause eye strain and require good vision. Another beneficial treatment is Botox injections for muscles that spasm creating pain. Some people, whose careers are in the spotlight, may choose any of the above therapies for their appearance as opposed to their health. They may also chose the dye their hair, get a tummy tuck, a face-lift, liposuction, or breast enhancement. New treatments that counter the effects of aging continue to be developed. And regardless of which school of thought you adhere to, you must remind yourself that all of these procedures are intended for your benefit. But it is important to balance a crucial health need with a service we chose simply for vanity's sake. It is also important to ensure that experienced medical professionals are performing any procedure.

Emotional health is also a crucial part of aging. It is important to be socially active and stay connected with family and friends. For those of us who are busy with careers and family, balance is the key to maintaining the physical and emotional health that will ensure continued and long-term independence. And remember, careers are important, but it is important to invest time and energy into our family and our friends, as they are our support group.

Sometimes unconditional friendships can be sorely tested. Sometimes the most conservative member our group will do something that we deem fool hearty without consulting our inner circle. But do we turn our backs on this friend? Do we talk behind their back or worse, pity them? What gives us this right? At what point in a true friendship are we there for any other purpose than to be a support or to provide a cushion if they fall? We need to remember that we are all getting older. We have no way of knowing what awaits us around the next corner. To live and let live is paramount in maintaining a friendship. Offer advice only when asked. And don't ask for advice unless you really mean it and are prepared to accept the advice we are offered.

Good communication creates a solid basis for any relationship. If we don't acknowledge and express feelings in our personal relationships we risk harboring anger and resentment over a possible misunderstanding. And this can lead to depression. Friendships allow us to share our thoughts and fears. Friends offer us insight from their perspective, which might help us to see important issues more clearly. True friends know that they cannot change our mind; they forgive us when we make mistakes and they admire us for being authentic individuals.

Just as our social life is important as we age, it is important to become reacquainted with ourselves, as individuals, and decide what it is that we really want out of life. Some thought provoking questions we might ask ourselves are: How do we perceive ourselves in the years to come? What are our fears over aging? What can we do right now that will have the most positive impact on our tomorrow? Coping with change is difficult no matter how old we are. It is important to focus on what is really important in life, to think about the things that we really enjoy. Lack of enjoyment can lead to aging and depression. Fun activities keep us vital and youthful. Perhaps there is an old hobby or activity that you once enjoyed. Even as we discover our limitations, as we age, we can continue to find enjoyment.

We direct our own destinies. If there is room for change it is entirely up to us. Life is meant to be lived, so get out there and claim your place in it. Whether it is physical or mental, try something new. When we embrace the thrill of life, we feel more alive. We look forward to its intimacy and linger in the sensuality of it. This can be experienced at any age, but it is up to us to reignite the spark. If we wait for someone else to do it for us, it might never happen. So if you are reading this, choose the spark that you want to reignite, put this book down and get out there and live your life!

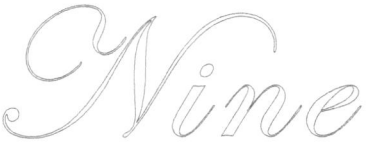

Eyes Wide Open

The current North American diet lacks essential enzymes, puts our bodies into an acid state, and leaves us prone to disease. This diet is high in processed and red meat, simple carbohydrates, refined sugars, and dairy. Chemicals are often used when processing these foods to lengthen shelf life. Processed meats are loaded with nitrates and nitrites. Dinner entrees contain refined carbohydrates, sugars, saturated fats, and preservatives. They are packaged in plastic and labeled 'Healthy Choice,' 'Lite,' '50% less fat,' '50% less sugar' and 'Low in saturated fats.' These are all buzz words which beg the question '50% less of what food value?' and 'Since when was any saturated fat good for me?' If we don't want to compromise our health by exposing ourselves to all of this, we need to turn our backs on what the food industry insists is good for us, and demand that safer, more nutritious products occupy shelf space at our local grocer.

We mindlessly zoom through the aisles, load up our grocery carts and hand over our hard-earned cash for food that is little better than toxic waste. We follow this by handing more hard-earned cash over to the pharmaceutical industry to cure our poorly nourished bodies. Our bodies are incredibly complex. They cannot be sustained on refined convenience foods. Cooking shouldn't be treated like a three-yard dash from the freezer to the microwave to the table. And bolting down a chemically laden, nuked, supposedly "Healthy Choice" meal is hardly what I would call meaningful time with the family. It is a toxic bullet that I avoid.

If you don't wish to load up your refrigerator and pantry with unhealthy food, my best advice to you is to keep your eyes wide open at the grocery store. Treat each aisle you pass through as if it were booby-trapped with toxic land mines, and that the way to get around them, and to make healthy choices for you and your family, is to read every label of the foods you select before putting them into your cart. When you pick processed, chemically laden, sugar loaded crap (and yes, it is crap) that the food industry actively promotes, you are really inviting the pharmaceutical industry to provide future interventions. It's best to be aware of what you are buying and to count every bad item as a nail in your coffin.

Your health is up to you. If you are the one doing the shopping and the cooking, your family's health is also up to you. When you really think about it, your choices have a far-reaching affect. The items that you put into your cart are what your grocery store manager stocks on his shelves. And these items, by virtue of taking up shelf space, also influence the shopping choices of others. But one person can make a huge difference. One simple request to a store manager for a product that really is healthy oftentimes gets results. And if you don't get satisfaction at the store level, you can always contact head office. Any good company wants to maintain customer satisfaction.

Being an advocate for change begins by complimenting a store manager for what he or she is doing right, before suggesting what would make it even better. An advocate also encourages friends to support positive change. Buy organic yourself and subtly encourage others to do likewise. And if you peel the plastic wrapping off the produce after it has been rung through the cash register, and ask that it be disposed of there, you will be subtly letting the manager know that plastic is harmful. Also, when inferior products are no longer being purchased, they will eventually be de-listed, as shelf space is valuable. Finally, if you exude good health and positive energy, as you go through the food aisles, others will notice, scan your cart, and note the differences between your choices and theirs. Simple actions speak louder than words; if you exude good health and demonstrate healthy choices, you, in essence, have said it all without uttering a word!

Bisphenol A (BPA)

Bisphenol A (BPA) is a chemical used in the production of plastics and resins. These plastics and resins have imploded the marketplace. BPA is used everywhere, including in products that we use daily. The list below is just *some* of the products that contain (BPA) this list is meant to enlighten you, and this is just a small list:

- Dental Composites
- Dental sealants
- Refillable beverage containers
- Protective linings in food cans
- Plastic Dinnerware
- Fungicides
- Antioxidant
- Flame Retardant
- Rubber chemical
- Polyvinyl Chloride Stabilizer
- Film, sheets, laminations
- Reinforced pipes
- Floorings
- Water main filters
- Enamels and varnishes
- Adhesives

- Artificial teeth
- Nail polish
- Electric insulators
- Automotive industry
- Technical Office equipment
- Machines
- Tools
- Electric appliances

Keeping in mind there is an overload of chemicals in food offered in the marketplace one is surprised to learn that there is added chemical in the packaging. Keep in mind even product labeled as organic when packaged in cans, plastic or cardboard have the ability to leech BPA into its' content if heated up in the originating package. Cans containing food have been found to be lined with an epoxy resin that contains BPA.

I still shudder at the thought of the plastic liners introduced into the marketplace in the 70's to replace glass bottles, these plastic liners that were filled with formula, inserted into plastic baby bottles and then into boiling water to warm for baby! This very product used to feed baby was toxic. Prenatal classes mandate is to teach parents to be how to safely prepare and look after baby upon arrival. In the 70's Prenatal Classes taught the two best choices offered to mothers were breastfeeding or bottle-feeding with unbreakable plastic bottles. To drive this point home was easy, they showed a picture of scar on an unfortunate baby's face resulting from a broken glass bottle in a baby's crib for everyone to see! A parent's guilt is heightened when they buy into the safer is better product, and then find out down the road the very product they believed safe was toxic. A baby that does not have the ability to choose for self has been introduced to toxins form the person they trusted the most. Like the introduction of new improved "BPA-free" soothers for baby!

Instantly panic erupts amongst those that chose soothers as a viable choice to prevent crooked teeth reeling with guilt knowing that they unwittingly introduced toxins to their baby since this new "BPA-free" product states so.

For years we drank from plastic bottles, thinking this to be the "superior choice" for many reasons, we knew water was healthier than soda pop and the plastic bottle added no more weight to the beverage than the actual beverage and if the child disposed of the plastic bottle we were not out any large amount of money. We also thought of the plastic bottle as good for the environment as it was recyclable. The plastic bottle was convenient to pack, you did not have to worry over the possibility of contaminated water while travelling outside of your region. Flashbacks for parents of how many school-aged children, toting plastic water bottles, lying on the sidelines exposed to the high temperatures of the sun! Surgical grade stainless steel is now the preferred choice, light weight and unbreakable and can be sterilized and re-used.

According to E. Huff, in 'Natural News,' (January 28, 2010), the Environmental Working Group (EWG) has found BPA in the umbilical cord blood of North American babies, for the first time in history. Nine out of ten samples tested positive for the chemical BPA. That's 90%! They also found 231 other chemicals. This shows that our continual exposure to chemicals is not going away. Studies show that BPA is dangerous in minimal levels. Low dose exposure, in developmental years, can actually cause more endocrine and reproductive problems than larger dose exposure later in life, due to the way the body recognizes the chemical. But keep in mind that BPA is legal in other countries and that we are a global market. As consumers, currently we need to read "BPA Free," to believe a product to be safe.

On one hand we are grateful in the transparency of information coming forward and we are grateful to see companies reacting swiftly in pulling products from their shelves and adopting better, safer products for their patrons and assuming the costs of lost revenue from these pulled products, but we are still left with the guilt on not being able to undo what we have unwittingly introduced to the innocent.

C.W. Randolph, M.D. and other leading scientists have found that BPA may impair our reproductive organs; that it may have adverse effects on tumors; that it can cause breast tissue development; and that it can impact prostate development by reducing sperm count. Imagine the heartache, in the years to come, when the outfall from BPA is finally understood in its entirety.

For many ignorance is bliss, for me knowledge is invaluable. I realize we as humans have contaminated our air, soils and oceans and the chicks are coming home to roost. I do what I can with what I have to work with. I know eating the raw live vegan lifestyle plays a large role on my internal system, the diet is rich in live enzymes and nutrients that boost my immunities to fight off the impurities that enter my system unwittingly. Stand back and assess how food is packaged refuse organic when it is packaged on Styrofoam trays enveloped in plastic, this mode of packaging is to convenience who? The retailer will say it is to guarantee you the shopper, that packaging this product assures the consumer that there is no chance of mix up between organic and nonorganic, when in fact they have exposed the organic product to toxins. We have a long way to go to educate the public and the retailer in food safety. It is wiser to know your source, buy direct, and bring your own cloth bags. When buying organics in stores that are stored loosely make sure you do rinse before consumption. When making baby food, process in a blender organic fresh product with a little water, the only two ingredients necessary, made fresh, right along with your own meal.

Again, be aware, intuition is primal!

> "Thank you for your kind and generous words regarding my participation in your wellness journey. The truth is you both have chosen and continue to choose the activities to obtain and maintain increasingly better health. That's the big power of your actions - real healthy results and outcomes! You are living the daily choices and activities that demonstrate the practical reality of healthy input gives healthy results."
> ~ Dr. J. William LaValley

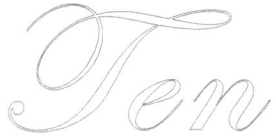

Menu Planners

Menu Planner, Week 1

Breakfast is the most important meal of the day, so enjoy your breakfast shake. It provides you with your daily requirement of fruits and vegetables in a single serving. Your soaked cereal groats provide a delicious source of excellent fibre as well. You are as limited in flavour as your imagination! Check out our recipe section.

Not all protein powders are created equal, so be careful when choosing protein powders for your morning shakes. Whey and soy-based protein powders are highly acidic and are very difficult for your body to process. The high temperature and chemicals needed to remove fat and carbohydrates, and to create a protein isolate in these products leaves behind toxic residues. Acid-based proteins, such as whey and soy, cause inflammation. This is the last thing a person needs when trying to lead an active lifestyle. Instead, try "Vega Complete Whole Food Health Optimizer." This product is an all-in-one natural plant-based formula. It contains 100% of the recommended daily intake of vitamins and minerals per serving. It is also rich in protein, fibre, omega-3 essential fatty acids, antioxidants and phytonutrients. It contains no common allergens, it is alkaline-forming and is easy to digest. Plant-based proteins protect against chronic diseases. They are also low in saturated fat and promote overall health. The protein shake is best consumed after a workout. Look for plant-based proteins such as hemp, spirulina, raw alfalfa juice, green pea protein, and raw sprouted rice, as choices in your plant-based protein powders.

Go Green Shake
Single Serving

Blend all ingredients until smooth, pour into tall glass. This will hold you until Lunch. Green combination drinks are healing, stabilizing and calming. And they have a relaxing, centering effect.

In Blender add:

- 1 tablespoon/15 ml of "Vega" Plant-Based Protein Powder
- 1 tablespoon/15 ml of *Multi Greens Plus*
- 1 tablespoon/15 ml of Ground Flax Seeds
- 1 teaspoon/5 ml of Spirulina
- 1 Banana
- 1 Kiwi
- 1 slice of Pineapple
- 1 cup/250 ml of purified water

Berry Good Morning Shake!
Single Serving

Blend all ingredients until smooth, pour into tall glass.

In Blender add:

- 1 tablespoon/15 ml of "Vega" Protein Powder
- 1 tablespoon/15 ml of *Multi Greens Plus*
- 1 tablespoon/15 ml of ground flax seed
- ½ cup/125 ml of blueberries
- ½ cup/125 ml of strawberries
- ½ cup/125 ml of raspberries

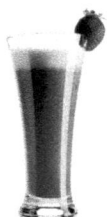

Multigrain Cereal
For Single Serving

Place the colander into a bowl or pot that is just a tad bigger than the colander. Cover with water and place a lid on it for 12 hours. In the morning, lift the colander out of bowl and let it drain thoroughly into the sink. Then place the soaked grains into a container as this will keep for four days in the fridge. Do not add more water to this mixture. In a glass jar with lid, put 1 cup/250 ml of walnuts and 1 teaspoon/5 ml of sea salt for an initial soak only. Drained the walnuts in the morning and add fresh water without salt.

It is now ready to eat, and provides great Fiber, Omega-3, and multiple nutrients.

*You may prefer to put the soaked, drained, cereal mix into a food processor, and then place it into a bowl, before topping it with your favourite fruit and almond milk.

In a large sieve/colander with tiny mesh holes put:

1 cup/250 ml of raw oat groats
1 cup/250 ml of raw buckwheat groats
1 cup/250 ml of raw barley

Place

½ cup/125 ml of prepared cereal into a bowl
1 teaspoon/5 ml of your choice: agave syrup, or #2 maple syrup, or raw honey, yacan syrup, or stevia
½ cup/125 ml of blueberries, or fruit of your choice
4 large walnuts cut up into pieces

Lunch: Lunch can be simply a salad, such as Quinoa, Bean Salad, or Green Salad. Use any combination of veggies and varieties of salad dressings. Again, check out the recipe section for ideas. In this single meal you will consume more than your daily vegetable requirements. And there is no need to ever eat the same salad twice. If you are packing salad to take to work, pack the salad dressing separately, so that the veggies don't go limp. Invest in good containers that do not leak and that are environmentally friendly; after all you are going greener!

Refer to "Recipes to get you started" for salad and dressing recipes.

Supper: Depending on your current progress or commitment level, I have two meal plan options to help you through the first week. The transitional meals are for those coming from diets that include a meat component. You may still have some remnants left to be eaten and choose to transition to raw live vegan slowly. You have the option to transition as slowly as you choose to, as this is a lifestyle and you have nobody to answer to but yourself. I also have Raw Live Vegan meals as an option for those that wish to transition more quickly. Again, go at your own pace, as there is no right or wrong way to transition into this program. And remember, the goal is 80%, so when you choose something that is not raw live vegan, count it as your 20% and you should remain guilt free.

Week 1 Transitional Meal 1

Stuffed Zucchini Boats
Single Serving or 2 Appetizers

Stuff ½ mixture in each zucchini half and top with goat cheese. There are many varieties of goat cheese - soft ripened, mozzarella and cheddar style. Bake at 350 F. for 25 minutes, and serve with a salad. See recipe section.

Wash and clean organic zucchini. Hollow out a bit of the centre and place in Food Processor and add the following ingredients to the right and lightly process:

   1 tablespoon/15 ml of olive oil
   2 tablespoons/30 ml of bread crumbs
   Dash of cayenne
   Dash of sea salt
   1 clove of finely chopped garlic

Week 1 Raw Live Vegan Meal 1
Teriyaki Vegetables with Pineapple Marinade
2 Servings or 4 Appetizers

One hour before company arrives prepare marinade for recipe.

In Food Processor add marinade ingredients:
1/2 cup/125 ml freshly juiced pineapple
1 tablespoon/15 ml of tamari
2 teaspoons/10 ml of agave syrup
2 teaspoons/10 ml sesame oil
2 teaspoons/10 ml of squeezed lemon juice
1 teaspoon/5 ml of chia (natural thickener)
1 teaspoon/5 ml of olive oil
1 teaspoon/5 ml mustard powder
1 teaspoon/5 ml of nama shoyu
1 teaspoon/5ml of chopped fine onion
1 teaspoon/5ml of sesame seeds
1 clove of fine chopped garlic
1/4 teaspoon/1 ml of grated ginger
Dash of cayenne pepper

Place marinade in dehydrator at 115 degrees F. for 1 hour to reduce.

As you are about to gather for the meal, rinse and chop artistically fresh raw organic vegetables, your choice, 1 cup each bok choy, broccoli, mushrooms, peppers and carrots and place into colander in sink. Pour almost-boiling water over vegetables allowing water to instantly pass over vegetables, through colander and down the drain. Vegetables will deepen in color yet maintain crispness. Place vegetables immediately into large bowl, pour marinade over warmed vegetables, toss lightly to evenly coat vegetables. Divide vegetables 4 plates. Top each plate with fresh raw organic pineapple chunks, fresh bean sprouts, 1 tablespoon of raw cashews and a dash of black caraway seeds. Try chop sticks instead of forks for utensils. Chop sticks are not only fun but will slow your eating pace and increase your attention on the food at hand allowing time to appreciate the incredible flavours!

Week 1 Transitional Meal 2
Poached Salmon & Spinach Salad

5 oz. cooked weight (skinless, boneless) salmon. Serve with steamed asparagus and grilled red pepper. Drizzle 1 teaspoon of olive oil over steamed vegetables and sprinkle with a dash of sea salt.

Spinach Salad:
   1 cup/250 ml spinach (packed)
   ½ cup/75 ml mushrooms
   ¼ cup /50 ml onions
   1 tablespoon/15 ml micro-planed goat's mozzarella

Dressing:
   2 teaspoon/10 ml olive oil
   2 teaspoon/10 ml white balsamic vinegar
   Juice from one orange
   1 teaspoon/5 ml sea salt

Week 1 Raw Live Vegan Meal 2
MOCKFish Stuffed Red Peppers
2 Servings

To make MOCKFish the only appliance required is the food processor, in processor add all of the ingredients listed to the right.

Mix all of the required ingredients in the food processor and add water slowly a bit at a time to get the desired texture. Remove stem from Red Pepper, cut in half creating two bowls, remove seeds and set aside on plates. Stuff each half with MOCKFish ingredients. Top with sprouted broccoli and serve with a spinach salad, see recipe in above "Transitional Meal 2."

   ¼ cup/50 ml of soaked and dried sunflower seeds
   ¼ cup/50 ml of soaked and dried almonds

¼ cup/50 ml of celery
¼ cup/50 ml of Spanish onion
2 tablespoons/30 ml fresh cilantro
2 tablespoons/30 ml fresh dill
1 clove of garlic
1 tablespoon/15 ml of micro-planed carrot
1 tablespoon/15 ml of dried arame (seaweed)
1 tablespoon/15 ml of fresh squeezed lime juice
1 teaspoon/5 ml of fresh chopped dill
½ teaspoon/2 ml of miso

Week 1 Transitional Meal 3

Carrot Ginger Soup with Waldorf Salad
2 Servings

Carrot Ginger Soup:

Sauté 6 carrots, in a tablespoon of olive oil, with 1/2 a medium onion and 1/2 stalk of celery, until soft. Continue to cook for 5 minutes. Place sautéed ingredients into Vita Mix Blender or Food Processor along with ingredients to the right:

1/2 teaspoon/5 ml of fresh ground ginger
2 cups/500 ml of organic vegetable broth
Zest of 1/2 lemon
Juice of 1/2 a lemon
Blend until smooth, pour into bowls
Top with ••• teaspoon/2 ml lime zest for garnish and serve!

• Enjoy soup with a Waldorf salad and top with Vinaigrette salad dressing; see recipe section.

Week 1 Raw Live Vegan Meal 3

Curry Carrot Soup with Lime & Waldorf Salad
Serves Two

In Vita Mix Blender add the ingredients to right:

- Enjoy with a fresh Waldorf Salad. Top with Vinaigrette salad dressing; see recipe section.

Juice of 6 carrots
1/2 stalk of sliced celery
1/2 a medium onion
1/2 cup/125 ml of macadamia nuts
1/3 cup/75 ml of coconut meat
Fresh squeezed juice from 1/2 lime
1 teaspoon/5 ml of curry paste

Blend at high for 2 minutes. You will see steam in a Vita Mix blender, but it will not heat above 115 degrees F. If you do not have Vita Mix Blender use any blender or food processor. Warm if you wish at 118 degrees Fahrenheit until ready to serve.

Garnish with 1/2 teaspoon/2 ml of lime zest.

Week 1 Transitional Meal 4

Grilled Chicken with Broccoli & Carrots
Single Serving

Grill or poach skinless, boneless organic chicken breast until tender. In a bowl of freshly steamed broccoli and carrot sticks add 1 teaspoon/5 ml of olive oil and a dash of sea salt and paprika, toss lightly to coat.

- See Recipe section for Salads and salad dressings.

Week 1 Raw Live Vegan Meal 4

MOCKchicken Salad

- See recipe section with recipe "Chicken Little."

Week 1 Transitional Meal 5

Veggie Spaghetti

Vegetarian Spaghetti Sauce with Whole Wheat Pasta or Brown Rice Pasta.

Cook until vegetables are tender
Store extra sauce in fridge. Pour 1 cup/250ml of sauce onto 1 cup/250 ml of whole wheat pasta. Serve with a simple green salad and a tablespoon of a vinaigrette salad.

Take 1- 28 oz. can of organic tomato sauce or organic fresh diced tomatoes mixed with water and heat on medium heat, then add:

    ½ cup/125 ml of chopped broccoli
    ¼ cup/50 ml of chopped spinach
    ½ small onion diced
    1 clove of garlic
    1 diced jalapeno pepper

Week 1 Raw Live Vegan Meal 5

Marinara on Zucchini Noodles

- See recipe section

Week 1 Transitional Meal 6
Steak and Blue Cheese Salad
Steak and Blue Cheese Salad:
> 3 oz. of grilled organic beef steak, medium rare, sliced ribbon thin
> 2 oz. of goat's blue cheese

Toss with:
> ½ head of organic romaine lettuce
> 1 cup/250 ml of organic greens
> 1 cup/250 ml of cherry tomatoes. sliced in half
> 1 cup/250 ml of chopped cucumber
> ¼ cup/50 ml of red pepper
> Dash of cayenne pepper

Top with:
> 2 tablespoons/30 ml of olive oil
> 2 tablespoons/30 ml of white wine vinegar
> 1 tablespoon/15 ml of Nama Shoyu
> Juice squeezed from 1 fresh lemon
> Sea salt and fresh ground pepper to taste. Enjoy!

Week 1 Raw Live Vegan Meal 6
Marinated Portobello Mushrooms with Salad Greens
- See recipe section.

Week 1 Transitional Meal 7
Baked Beans and Coleslaw
Heat and serve with Cole Slaw.

398 ml can of organic black beans.

Cole Slaw
In bowl add:

 1 cup/250 ml of shredded carrot
 1 cup/250 ml of shredded cabbage
 In another bowl whisk:
 1 tablespoon/15 ml of egg free mayonnaise
 1 tablespoon/15 ml of white wine vinegar
 1 tablespoon/15 ml of soy milk
 Dash of cayenne pepper
 Dash of sea salt.

Toss with shredded carrot and cabbage.

Week 1 Raw Live Vegan Meal 7
Quinoa Salad with "the Works"
- See recipe section.

Transitional version would be 2 cans of organic bean medley to cooked Quinoa.

Snacks

Between meals, feel free to blend up some salsa to dip veggie sticks into. Or juice vegetables for an invigorating drink. Refer to the recipe section for ideas. If you are really hungry, try a hummus dip with veggie sticks.

Evening Meal Information while Transitioning

As you begin to transition from an acidic diet (meat protein based) to an alkaline diet (plant protein based), you can still eat 3 ounces of organic chicken or red meat (hopefully organic), or 5 ounces of fish for supper. Your meat can be roasted, poached or grilled, but never fried. You can have your choice of 1/2 - 1 cup/125-250 mL of cooked brown rice, or whole wheat pasta, or brown rice pasta or a medium baked potato with skin, or medium sweet potato or 1 cup of squash. You can have unlimited steamed vegetables or salad greens, with 1 tablespoon of cold pressed olive oil, a dash of sea salt and pepper, and a squeeze of lemon or lime. You must adhere to these limitations at supper for week 1. If you must have cheese, choose goat cheese products such as goat mozzarella, goat's feta, or goat's cheddar are recommended. Refer to the Allowable Food Lists and choose as many foods from this list as you can for your raw vegan breakfasts and lunches. For supper, if you refer to the pH chart you will see the wisest choices on the alkaline side of the chart.

Beverages

There are many great teas, on the market today, that I have found helpful for keeping me satisfied between meals. These include chocolate chai tea, mint tea, ginger tea, orange tea, and liquorice spice tea, to name a few. Mineral water, with the juice of half of a lemon in it or more, and a sweetener such as stevia will also hold you over. I quite enjoy a cup of hot green tea at breakfast. I add fresh lemon and stevia to the leftover tea, and store it in the fridge, for iced tea later in the day. If you must have coffee, it should be organic with one teaspoon of stevia to alkalize it. Again check out our recipe section.

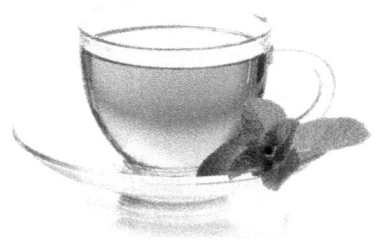

Week 2, What To Prepare For!

During Week 2 you will be trying to incorporate more meatless suppers, so stock up on your essentials from your allowable food lists. Also, refer to storage and shelf life of said items. Most items can be safely stored for longer periods in the freezer. I prefer to buy fresh and buy often. Slowly but surely, we will become accustomed to making pizza shells from our raw version of bread, raw mashed potato using cauliflower, and jicama to imitate rice. Start collecting some raw vegan recipes and have fun!

Going raw might seem like a formidable task when you concentrate only on its' limitations. For starters, get used to this site. Check out the food lists and then shop for what you need to get started. Although the goal is 80%, you will call the shots as to how fast you reach that goal. You may start off at a 50% ratio, or do raw live vegan for 3 days a week. It's your choice, you set the pace. My transition took a few months. Knowing that you have a goal of becoming a true raw live vegan person, 20% of your food choices can come from items such as meat or sweets. Your transition should be a place of calm. Search through recipe books and check out your local markets to see what's available. This is a whole new lifestyle that will deliver you to a level of fitness you never dreamed possible. When we think, 'no processed foods, no refined sugars, no dairy, no refined carbohydrates', we wonder what is left? The answer is 'Plenty.' There is a huge variety of good foods to choose from: vegetables, fruits, legumes, nuts, seeds and grains.

The best place to start transitioning is with Breakfast. If you start the day off right, you will tend to want to keep up the momentum, especially when you see and feel the benefits of the changes you are making. Go to our recipe section for some great ideas for Breakfast. We are too conditioned to pulling a box of cereal out of the cupboard and adding milk and sugar to it. You will be amazed at what real, tasty, raw, nutritious cereal tastes like. When we dwell on eliminating meat, fish, poultry, eggs, and dairy, the first question we ask is 'what is the source of protein on this program?' The answer is plant-based foods such vegetables, legumes, nuts, seeds and mushrooms. These foods can be digested and processed easily by the GI tract and will transform your health and physical body at a rapid pace.

Before you start the program, consider any medical conditions you might have. If you are dealing with medical issues involving the GI tract, you will need to correct this first, with help from your doctor. But, if you enjoy good health, you can choose how fast you transition from your current lifestyle to the raw live vegan lifestyle. Remember the goal is 80% raw live vegan. Think of saving the remaining 20% to enjoy the foods you simply can't live without, without feeling guilty. Bean salad is an easy meal. Beans are a great source of protein and are very satisfying. I pack a bean salad when I am working erratic shifts. Beans fit well in the vegan program, but to become edible they must be cooked. To compromise, consider adding live sprouts to bring it up a notch. Also, add a variety of raw veggies. Bean salad is a great transitional recipe. Adding raw sprouts will train your taste buds. Eventually, you may leave out the cooked beans altogether, or enjoy them as part of your other 20%. Take time to adjust. The bonus comes when you transition from cooked beans to live sprouts and experience less flatulence!

Since going raw, I am never without food. My pantry and freezer are stocked with plenty of ingredients. These are ingredients that are in their natural state, and ready to be transformed into delectable healthy dishes. The best part of this program is that you can adjust the recipes to suit your own personal tastes. I practice the raw live vegan lifestyle 80% at home. I also do so when traveling, but this is a personal choice. It is just a way of life, second nature now. The result has been that I have achieved optimum health and have never felt better in my life!

Menu Planner, Week 2

For week 2, your breakfast and lunch choices will be the same as for week 1. This will help you to adjust to the program. In future weeks, you will be introduced to dehydrated breakfast breads, nut yogurts and more. But, nothing is more nutritionally complete than your morning breakfast shake and prepared groats. Also, salads are as limited as your imagination. Concentrate on organic this week with your foods. Most recipes featured on this site are for two people. If you find the servings small, simply increase the quantity of ingredients as you curb your appetite. Ditto if you are preparing meals for three or more. These healthy food choices will boost your energy and allow you to actively participate in any physical activity of your choice.

Be careful when selecting protein powders, as they are not all created equal. Whey and soy-based protein powders are highly acidic and work against you, as they are very difficult for your body to process. In order to create the protein isolate, chemicals and high temperatures are used to remove fat and carbohydrates. This process leaves toxic residues. Acid-based proteins also cause inflammation. This is the last thing a person needs when trying to lead an active lifestyle. Instead, try the "Vega" Brand Complete Whole Food Health Optimizer. This is an all-in-one, natural, plant-based formula, which provides 100 percent of the recommended daily intake (RDI) of vitamins and minerals per serving. It is rich in protein, fibre, omega-3 essential fatty acids (EFAs), antioxidants, and phytonutrients. It contains no common allergens, it is alkaline-forming and is easy to digest. Plant-based proteins protect against chronic diseases, are low in saturated fat, and promote overall health. Look for plant-based proteins such as hemp, spirulina, raw alfalfa juice, green pea protein, and raw sprouted rice, as choices for your plant-based protein powders. And remember that the protein shake is best consumed after a workout.

Go Green Shake
Single Serving

Blend all ingredients until smooth and pour into a tall glass. Enjoy!

This will hold you until Lunch. Green combination drinks are healing, stabilizing and calming, as they have a relaxing, centering effect.

In Blender add:

- 1 tablespoon/15 ml of "Vega" Plant-Based Protein Powder
- 1 tablespoon/15 ml of *Multi Greens Plus*
- 1 tablespoon/15 ml of Ground Flax Seeds
- 1 teaspoon/5 ml of Spirulina
- 1 banana
- 1 kiwi
- 1 slice of Pineapple
- 1 cup/250 ml of purified water

Berry Good Morning Shake!
Single Serving

Blend all ingredients until smooth, pour into tall glass. Enjoy!

In Blender add:

- 1 tablespoon/15 ml of "Vega" Plant-Based Protein Powder
- 1 tablespoon/15 ml of *Multi Greens Plus*

1 tablespoon/15 ml of Ground Flax Seed
1/2 cup/125 ml of blueberries
1/2 cup/125 ml of strawberries
1/2 cup/125 ml of raspberries

Multigrain Cereal
For Single Serving

Place colander into a bowl or pot that is just a tad larger, then cover with water and place a lid on it for 12 hours. In the morning, lift the colander out of the bowl and let the grains drain thoroughly into the sink. Then place the grains into a container; they will keep for four days in the fridge. Do not add more water to this mix.

In a glass jar with a lid put 1 cup/250 ml of walnuts. Fill the jar with water and 1 teaspoon/5 ml of sea salt, for an initial soak only. This will be drained in the morning and fresh water will be added without the salt. Soak for 5 days only. Remember, the shelf life of soaked walnuts is 5 days, so never soak more walnuts than you can eat over this time period.

*You may prefer to put soaked, drained, cereal mix into a food processor to blend, before placing it into your cereal bowl and topping it with your favorite fruit and almond milk.

In a large sieve/colander with tiny mesh holes put:

1 cup/250 ml of raw oat groats
1 cup/250 ml of raw buckwheat groats
1 cup/250 ml of raw barley

Place:

½ cup/125 ml of prepared cereal into a bowl
1 teaspoon/5 ml of your choice: agave syrup, or #2 maple syrup, or raw honey, yacan syrup, or stevia
½ cup/125 ml of blueberries, or fruit of your choice
4 large walnuts cut up into pieces

This is now ready to eat, great fiber, with Omega-3 and multiple nutrients.

Lunch: can be simply a salad, such as Quinoa, Bean Salad, or Green Salad. Use any combination of veggies and varieties of salad dressings. Again, check out the recipe section for ideas. In this single meal you will consume more than your daily vegetable requirements. And there is no need to ever eat the same salad twice. If you are packing salad to take to work, pack the salad dressing separately, so that the veggies don't go limp. Invest in good containers that do not leak and that are environmentally friendly; after all you are going greener!

Supper: You may still have some remnants left to be eaten and choose to transition to raw live vegan slowly. You have the option to transition as slowly as you choose to, as this is a lifestyle and you have nobody to answer to but yourself. I also have Raw Live Vegan meals as an option for those that wish to transition more quickly. Again, go at your own pace, as there is no right or wrong way to transition into this program. And remember, the goal is 80%, so when you choose something that is not raw live vegan, count it as your 20% and you should remain guilt free.

Week 2 Raw Live Vegan Meal 1

Sweet and Sour Chinese Vegetables - RAW
Marinade - In a casserole dish add:

Juice from one pineapple
Juice from one lime
2 tablespoons/30 ml of Tamari
2 tablespoons/30 ml of Braggs amino acids
4 cloves of minced garlic
1 tablespoon/15 ml of sucanat (dehydrated cane sugar)
1 tablespoon/15 ml of tahini
1 tablespoon/15 ml of sesame oil
1 tablespoon/15 ml of hemp oil
1 teaspoon/5 ml of grated ginger
1/2 cup/125 ml of pre-soaked cashews (see soaking chart)

Place casserole dish into dehydrator for 2 hours, this will serve to reduce and meld the flavours to pour over your veggies.

Vegetables- In large colander add:

1 cup/250 ml of snow peas
1 cup/250 ml of carrots, cut into match sticks
1 cup/250 ml of diced celery
1 cup/250 ml of broccoli florettes
1/2 cup/125 ml of broccoli tender stems, finely chopped
1/4 cup/50 ml of onion

Pour *almost boiling water* over the vegetables while in the colander. This prevents the vegetables from sitting in *almost boiling water* for too long and killing important enzymes.

Divide vegetables into serving dishes, top with chopped fresh pineapple, pour marinade on top, and sprinkle with sesame seeds and broccoli sprouts. Then serve.

Week 2 Raw Live Vegan Meal 2

Vegetable Kebabs
On skewers arrange, in any fashion, in a casserole dish:

4 cherry tomatoes
1 cubed zucchini
½ head of broccoli
½ head of cauliflower
2 carrots diced
4 crimini mushrooms
Onion cut in half (use in shell shape to skewer)

Marinade - In food processor blend:

¼ cup/50 ml tamari
¼ cup/50 ml hemp oil
3 red chili peppers
1 tablespoon/15 ml of agave syrup
1 tablespoon/15 ml of psyllium

1 teaspoon/5 ml of sea salt
1 teaspoon/5 ml of basil

Pour marinade over skewered vegetables and marinade overnight in refrigerator. Place casserole dish into the dehydrator to dehydrate for 24 hours at 105 degrees.

Week 2 Transitional Meal 3
Black Bean Soup

Start the Vita Mix blender on a low setting, going from 1-10 plunging the vegetables down. Turn to high and blend for 5 more minutes, until steam comes out of vent. Serve with spicy flax crackers!

In a Vita Mix blender place:

>14 oz/398 ml of organic black beans, rinsed and drained
>2 cups/500 ml of organic vegetable juice
>2 cups/500 ml of chopped organic carrots
>1 cup/250 ml of chopped organic celery
>1 cup/250 ml of organic red pepper
>1 cup/250 ml of organic green pepper
>3 tablespoons/45 ml of chopped jalapeno peppers
>1 clove of garlic
>1 teaspoon/5 ml of sea salt
>1 teaspoon/5 ml of cumin

Week 2 Raw Live Vegan Meal 4
Spiced Lentils Caribbean Style
Sauce - In small bowl add:

>2 tablespoons of cold pressed olive oil
>Juice from one lime
>½ teaspoon/5 ml of thyme
>¼ teaspoon/1 ml of nutmeg
>¼ teaspoon/1 ml of allspice
>¼ teaspoon/1 ml of cinnamon
>2 teaspoons/10 ml of sea salt
>Grinds of Fresh black pepper

Salad - In large bowl add:

2 cups/500 ml of sprouted lentils
2 cloves of finely chopped garlic
½ teaspoon/2 ml of freshly grated ginger
½ cup/125 ml of finely chopped onions
¾ cup/200 ml of chopped green pepper
¾ cup/200 ml of chopped red pepper

Add sauce to the top of the bean salad and top with chopped cilantro. Enjoy!

Week 2 Raw Live Vegan Meal 5

Thai Special RAW
In a large salad bowl add:

2 cups/500 ml of sprouted lentils
1 cup of grated jicama, or cauliflower chopped into the texture of rice
½ cup/125 ml of pre-soaked sunflower seeds
½ cup/125 ml of chopped scallions
¼ cup/50 ml of green pepper
¼ cup/50 ml of red pepper
3 jalapeno peppers cut into thin rings

With a hand blender, blend dressing ingredients and pour dressing onto salad ingredients and let marinate in fridge for at least one hour before serving. Serve on a kale leaf, chopped kale, or a bed of baby spinach leaves. Top with radish sprouts.

Dressing:

½ cup/125 ml of olive oil
¼ cup/50 ml of rice wine vinegar
1 teaspoon/5 ml of tahini sauce
½ teaspoon/2 ml of sesame oil
½ teaspoon/2 ml of tamari sauce
½ teaspoon/2 ml of sea salt

Week 2 Transitional Meal 6
Squash Stew
In a large pot add:

1 28 oz/796 ml can of organic diced tomatoes
1 10 oz/198 ml can of organic vegetable broth
1 19 oz/398 ml can of organic kidney beans, rinsed and drained
1 cup/250 ml of water

In a sauté pan add:

3 medium onions diced
1 cup/250 ml of celery diced
3 cloves of /10 ml of cumin
1 tablespoon/15 ml of safflower oil

Sauté 1 small Spanish onion until softened and then in sauté pan with 1 tablespoon of olive oil until tender, then add to large pot.

Add for your preferred taste:

Grinds of sea salt
Grinds of cayenne pepper
Srirachi sauce

Cook at medium heat for 45 minutes. Then add the chopped squash from one butternut squash and cook for 20 minutes more. This prevents the squash from going to mush. Enjoy!

Week 2 Raw Live Vegan Meal 7
Peanut Miso Noodles RAW

This recipe is featured on the back of the package. How Nice is that!

In a serving dish add:

12 oz/340 g package of Kelp Noodles, cut to desired length
Add chopped veggies:
Red pepper

Green pepper
Onions
Carrots
Snow peas
½ cup/125 ml of pre-soaked cashews

Sauce:

1 part miso paste
2 parts ground peanuts or organic peanut butter
Add water to desired consistency of sauce
1 tablespoon/15 ml of sucanat (dehydrated cane sugar)
Dash of sesame oil and rice wine vinegar

I order my sea noodles, by the box, from Sea Tangle Noodles. They arrive in 12 oz packets, packed in sea water. They do not require refrigeration until the packet is opened. Find them online at: www.kelpnoodles.com.

Menu Planner, Week 3

In preparation for Week 3, be prepared for total Raw Live Vegan Recipes. If you feel the need to continue to transition slowly, add fish or organic poultry or goat cheese products. We will continue to feature a weekly live video of a recipe prepared in the Raw Live Vegan kitchen. Remember, the first take is the final take; good for a chuckle, I'm sure.

On week 3, continue to enjoy your breakfast shakes. Vary your fruit, but always include your *Greens Plus*, plant-based pea-protein powder, ground flax and spirulina. This is the best way to start your day! Enjoy some prepared raw groats. Remember, you can sweeten them with maple syrup #2, yacan syrup, agave syrup, raw honey, or sucanat with almond milk. I like a dash of cinnamon too. We will do breakfast breads soon, on future episodes. Variety is the spice of life. For Lunch, continue with unlimited varieties in salads, by adding small amounts of fruits and seeds to your other salad ingredients. Never be bored and never be hungry!

Most recipes serve two people. But, feel free to make larger batches for leftovers or to have a little extra if you are hungry. Remember, it's best to curb your appetite, gently, on high quality foods that are designed to energize you and to allow you to become more active.

Be careful when selecting protein powders, as they are not all created equal. Whey and soy-based protein powders are highly acidic and work against you, as they are very difficult for your body to process. In order to create the protein isolate, chemicals and high temperatures are used to remove fat and carbohydrates. This process leaves toxic residues. Acid-based proteins also cause inflammation. This is the last thing a person needs when trying to lead an active lifestyle. Instead, try the "Vega" Brand Complete Whole Food Health Optimizer. This is an all-in-one, natural, plant-based formula, which provides 100 percent of the recommended daily intake (RDI) of vitamins and minerals per serving. It is rich in protein, fibre, omega-3 essential fatty acids (EFAs), antioxidants, and phytonutrients. It contains no common allergens, it is alkaline-forming and is easy to digest. Plant-based proteins protect against chronic diseases, are low in saturated fat, and promote overall health. Look for plant-based proteins such as hemp, spirulina, raw alfalfa juice, green pea protein, and raw sprouted rice, as choices for your plant-based protein powders. And remember that the protein shake is best consumed after a workout.

Go Green Shake
Single Serving - see previous section.

Berry Good Morning Shake
Single Serving - see previous section.

Multigrain Cereal
For Single Serving - see previous section.

Lunch: can be simply a salad, such as Quinoa, Bean Salad, or Green Salad. Use any combination of veggies and varieties of salad dressings. Again, check out the recipe section for ideas. In this single meal you will consume more than your daily vegetable requirements. And there is no need to ever eat the same salad twice. If you are packing salad to take to work, pack the salad dressing separately, so that the veggies don't go limp. Invest in good containers that do not leak and that are environmentally friendly; after all you are going greener!

Supper: You may still have some remnants left to be eaten and choose to transition to raw live vegan slowly. You have the option to transition as slowly as you choose to, as this is a lifestyle and you have nobody to answer to but yourself. I also have Raw Live Vegan meals as an option for those that wish to transition more quickly. Again, go at your own pace, as there is no right or wrong way to transition into this program. And remember, the goal is 80%, so when you choose something that is not raw live vegan, count it as your 20% and you should remain guilt free.

Week 3 Raw Live Vegan Meal Day 1

Best Curry Noodles
Rinse and leave in a colander to drain, 1 package of sea kelp noodles.

In a blender add the following ingredients:

    1 cup/250 ml of water
    1/2 cup/125 ml of macadamia nuts
    1/4 cup/50 ml of coconut meat
    1 tablespoon/15 ml of curry paste
    2 teaspoons/10 ml of chili paste
    1/2 teaspoon/2 ml of sea salt

Blend until you achieve a thick, rich, creamy texture. Test-taste for desired flavour.

Divide sea kelp noodles into two bowls.

On top of noodles add the following ingredients:

1/4 cup/50 ml kernels of corn
1/2 cup/125 ml each of finely diced green, red, and orange peppers
1/4 cup/50 ml of finely diced celery

Pour the rich, creamy sauce on top of the noodles and vegetables. Sprinkle with a dash of cayenne pepper. Enjoy!

Week 3 Raw Live Vegan Meal Day 2

Veggie Nut Burger

Add to a food processor and process nuts that have been pre-soaked for 3 hours (refer to Soaking Chart). The nuts do not have to be dried, as we will be adding liquid to them.

2 cups/500 ml of raw almonds
2 cups/500 ml of raw sunflower seeds
2 cups/500 ml of raw walnuts
2 cups/500 ml of ground flax seeds

Place processed nuts into a large bowl, set aside.

In a food processor add the following ingredients:

3 cups/750 ml of mushrooms
1 yellow onion
2 cups/500 ml of chopped celery
3 carrots
1 red pepper
1 zucchini

Add the processed vegetables to the large bowl of processed nuts.

Also add to the above mixture:

Cloves of 1 whole garlic bulb, finely chopped
1/2 bunch of parsley leaves, finely chopped
1/2 bunch of tarragon leaves, finely chopped
1/2 bunch of cilantro leaves, finely chopped

In a small bowl add:

1/2 cup/125 ml of flax oil
1 ½ cup/375 ml of nama shoyu
1/2 cup/125 ml of Braggs Liquid Soy, all purpose flavouring

Mix the above liquids with a hand blender and add to the large bowl.

Mix the large batch well. Test-taste to see if anything is missing.

Spoon it onto teflon coated racks and shape into patties or small round balls, to make mock meat balls (great for dipping). Dehydrate at 105 degrees Fahrenheit for 12 hours on one side. Remove from the teflon coated racks and flip onto the wire racks, without teflon, and continue to dehydrate for another 12-18 hours, depending on how dry you want them to be. What I like about this recipe is that the nut burgers are savory. You can 'grab and go,' knowing that you have your protein, your veggies and high quality fibre, all in one. Enjoy on Herbed Onion Bread or in Marinara Sauce on your favourite veggie noodles!

Week 3 Raw Live Vegan Meal Day 3

Nori Rolls

Place a nori sheet on top of a bamboo sushi mat. Spread the olive tapenade into a narrow row down the narrow end of the nori sheet. Lay thin slivers of vegetables down the centre on top of the tapenade. Be sure to leave some colourful vegetable sticks sticking out at each end. These will provide a decorative centre and make a nice display on your dish. Roll tightly. When you get to the last inch of the empty nori sheet, dip a finger into the rice wine vinegar and rub it lightly along the end of the nori sheet, before completing the roll. Rest the weight of the roll along the edge to seal. I cut each end of the nori roll longer than the ones in the middle, so that they stand out in the centre of the display dish. Serve with a small serving dish of wasabi paste and a small serving dish of nama shoyu. Enjoy!

- Hint: use a sharp, cerated knife for slicing the nori roll. I dip my knife into fresh water before each cut. I also wipe any residue off the knife to be sure that the blade is smooth before dipping and cutting. This way you will not tear the nori sheet when you cut through it. Refer to my video as a visual aid for this recipe.

* Old style mustard has the seeds visible in the mix.

Olive Tapenade filling for Nori Rolls
In a food processor process:

1 cup/250 ml of olives
1 cup/250 ml of sunflower seeds
2 tablespoons/30 ml of minced garlic
2 tablespoons/30 ml of minced scallions
2 tablespoons/30 ml of old style mustard*
2 tablespoons/30 ml of olive oil
2 tablespoons/30 ml of nama shyu
2 tablespoons/30 ml of fresh minced dill
2 tablespoons/30 ml of fresh minced cilantro

Set the above mixture aside.

Slice into long match stick slivers:

1 red pepper
1 carrot
1 cucumber
1 avocado

Set slivered vegetables aside.

Pour into a small finger bowl 1 tablespoon of rice wine vinegar. This is used to seal the outer edge of the nori rolls. Set aside

Week 3 Raw Live Vegan Meal Day 4

Corn Chowder

In Vita Mix Blender, blend all ingredients until steam comes out of the lid of Blending jar. Pour into bowls. Store any remaining chowder in the fridge; it will keep for 4 days. Corn chowder can also be frozen for longer storage, if desired. Enjoy!

In a blender put:

6 cups of fresh corn nibblets
2 ½ cups/625 ml of water
1/2 cup/125 ml of pre-soaked macadamia nuts
2 teaspoons/10 ml of sea salt
1/2 teaspoon/2 ml of cayenne pepper
Blend at a high speed in a Vita

Week 3 Raw Live Vegan Meal Day 5

Veggie Pizza with Nut Cheese

Nut Cheese - In a food processor add:

1 cup/250 ml of pre-soaked sunflower seeds
Juice of one lemon
2 cloves of garlic
1 teaspoon/5 ml of sea salt

Water for desired consistency

Introduce the water slowly, adding a little at a time until satisfied with the texture and taste, then blend. If you wish, warm in a dehydrator at 105 degrees Fahrenheit for half an hour. Enjoy!

Tomato Paste - In a blender add:

1 cup of sun-dried tomatoes
1/2 cup/125 ml of olive oil
1/2 cup/125 ml of nama shoyu
1/4 cup/50 ml of Braggs soy flavouring
1/4 cup/50 ml of apple cider vinegar with mother

1/4 fresh squeezed lemon
4 cloves of garlic
2 tablespoons/30 ml of chopped oregano
2 tablespoons/30 ml of chopped cilantro
1 teaspoon/5 ml of sea salt

Spread the tomato paste onto Herbed Onion Bread shaped into triangles. Top with your choice of sliced vegetables, such as olives, mushrooms, or green and yellow peppers. Top the sliced vegetables with Nut Cheese.

- See recipe section.

Week 3 Raw Live Vegan Meal Day 6

Kale & Broccoli with Tahini Sauce

In a large colander, add cut up kale leaves, with the stems removed, and cut up broccoli heads and stems. These should all be cut up into bite-sized pieces. Set the colander into the sink, rinse with water, and leave to drain.

You can massage kale in the fist of your hands by squeezing leaves in hand continually until supple, and just rinse your broccoli if you do not want to flash steam. Or take a kettle of hot water, not boiling, and pour it over the kale/broccoli mixture in a colander, allowing the hot water to pour through. Place this warmed mixture into the large bowl of finely chopped vegetables. Pour on the tahini sauce and toss until everything is well coated. Divide into two bowls and top with sprouted mung beans.

This meal is my personal favourite. My husband makes it for me and it tastes just as wonderful each time. I hope you enjoy it as much as I do!

In a large bowl add:

1/4 of yellow onion diced fine
4 crimini mushrooms, finely diced
8 large walnuts, chopped into small pieces

Tahini Sauce - In a blender add:

Juice from 1 orange
1/2 teaspoon/2 ml of sesame oil
1 ½ tablespoons/20 ml of tahini
2 tablespoons/30 ml of cold pressed olive oil
2 tablespoons/30 ml of white balsamic vinegar
1 tablespoon/15 ml of miso

Blend and set aside.

Week 3 Raw Live Vegan Meal Day 7

Veggie Fries Combination Platter

Brush a thin coat of olive oil onto the sweet potato and zucchini. The avocado is moist enough to retain its coating.

Place coated vegetables onto a teflon-coated dehydrator rack and dehydrate for 1 hour at 118 degrees Fahrenheit. Enjoy with your favorite salad, or perhaps it will be a fun finger food, with salsa, vegetables and hummus, and flax crackers. Whatever the occasion, enjoy!

1 avocado, thinly sliced into thin wedges
1 small sweet potato, cut into French Fry shape
1 zucchini, with the centre row of seeds discarded, cut into French Fry shapes

Coat vegetables in the following blended, dry ingredients:

½ cup/125 ml of ground flax seeds
1 tablespoon/15 ml of nutritional yeast
2 teaspoons/10 ml of chili powder
2 teaspoons/10 ml of dried minced garlic (good for added crunch)
2 teaspoons/10 ml of cumin

2 teaspoons/10 ml of garam masala
2 teaspoons/10 ml of sea salt

Food Preparation, Timing & Organizing

Always plan meals the day before.

You will get into the pattern of having plenty of crackers made ahead as they store well. You will have plenty of nut burgers made ahead and frozen. You will want to have lots of breakfast breads made ahead too. You will become accustomed to checking the fridge for how much cereal groats and soaked nuts are on the shelf before you have to make more. When choosing a recipe check out the ingredient list, see if the recipe requires soaked nuts or seeds as an ingredient. How long will that nut or seed have to be soaked. Knowing this ahead of time is key for success in meal prep. I tend to prepare triple recipes on items that are used and enjoyed a lot, like crackers, vegan burgers, breads or cookies. These items can be frozen and defrost quickly for quick meal prep when days get hectic. Survey the fridge at night thinking ahead to next day before calling it a night. My freezer has been transformed to back up storage for grains nuts and seeds, over on top of what my pantry holds. I am conscientious of how much "Vega" protein powder, *Greens Plus* powder, spirulina powder, and fresh/frozen fruit I have on hand as our Go Go Green Shake is a staple every morning. An ongoing grocery list is handy to refer to what item you are getting low on, I add to this list when I hit the half gone point. Items I have not been able to purchase due to unavailability, I make sure to add to next list so it does not get forgotten totally! Learn to delegate and include family members or invited guests in the food preparation as this is quality time spent together! You will find that as you continue eating and reaping the benefits of this lifestyle other family members and friends are going to want to snack a little on what you are eating and before you know it, you have a house full of converts wanting what it is you eat. At this point is when you transition the grocery budget from the processed breads and crackers to more whole grains and nuts and triple your recipes to accommodate the new toll on your "good food!"

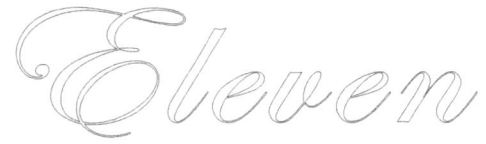

Recipes

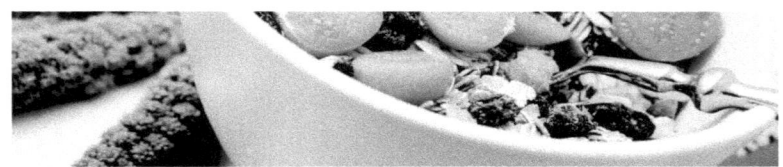

Breakfast Ideas

SOAK IT UP! Multigrain Cereal

Place colander in a bowl or pot that is just a tad bigger, then cover with water and place a lid on it for 12 hours! In the morning, lift colander out of bowl and let drain thoroughly in sink. Then place in container as this will keep for four days in fridge. Do not add water to this mix anymore. In a glass jar with lid put 1 cup of walnuts, 1 tsp of sea salt for initial soak only, this will be drained in morning and each day thereafter fresh water will be added to walnuts without the sea salt for the four days it's stored in the refrigerator.

The way cereal is really meant to taste! Great! Ready to eat, great Fiber, Omega-3, and multiple nutrients!

TIP You may prefer to put soaked, drained cereal mix in food processor for a porridge like consistency. Place soaked cereal mix on dehydrator rack for 2 hours to make a crunchy cereal.

Top cereal with your favorite fruit and almond milk. Make this your own version!

In a large sieve/colander with tiny mesh holes add the following ingredients:

 1 cup/250 mL of raw oat grouts
 1 cup/250 mL of raw buckwheat grouts
 1 cup/250 mL of raw barley

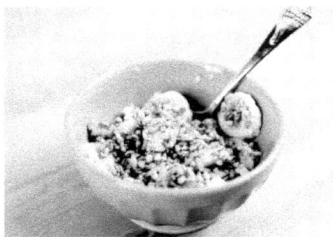

For Single Serving:

 Place 1/2 cup/125 mL of prepared cereal in bowl
 1 teaspoon/5 mL of your choice: agave syrup, #2 maple syrup, raw honey, yacan syrup, or stevia
 1/2 cup/125 mL of blueberries, or fruit of your choice
 4 large walnuts cut up into pieces

Cinnamon Apple Crunch

Pre- soak raw barley, oat groats and buckwheat groats in equal amounts the night before. Top cereal mix with water and soak overnight. In morning rinse very well leaving in colander until no more water is coming out. Store in fridge in sealed container for four days or dehydrate and store in pantry if crispy cereal is preferred.

 1/2 cup/125 mL of mixed presoaked groats
 1/2 cup/125 mL of chopped crisp granny smith apple
 1 tablespoon/15 mL of chopped pre-soaked almonds
 1 teaspoon/5 mL of agave syrup
 1 teaspoon/5 mL of cinnamon

Blueberrilicious Cereal

Pre- soak raw barley, oat groats and buckwheat groats in equal amounts the night before. Top cereal mix with water and soak overnight. In morning rinse very well leaving in colander until no more water is coming out. Store in fridge in sealed container for four days or dehydrate and store in pantry if crispy cereal is preferred.

> 1/2 cup/125 mL of mixed presoaked groats
> 1/4 cup/60 mL of wild blueberries
> 4 whole pre-soaked walnuts
> 1 tablespoon/15 mL of #2 maple syrup

Bananarama Cereal

Pre- soak raw barley, oat groats and buckwheat groats in equal amounts the night before. Top cereal mix with water and soak overnight. In morning rinse very well leaving in colander until no more water is coming out. Store in fridge in sealed container for four days or dehydrate and store in pantry if crispy cereal is preferred.

> 1/2 cup/125 mL of mixed presoaked groats
> 1 banana chopped
> 1 tablespoon/15 mL of cacao nibs
> 1 teaspoon/5 mL of sucanat

Strawberry Sunshine Groats

Pre- soak raw barley, oat groats and buckwheat groats in equal amounts the night before. Top cereal mix with water and soak overnight. In morning rinse very well leaving in colander until no more water is coming out. Store in fridge in sealed container for four days or dehydrate and store in pantry if crispy cereal is preferred.

1/2 cup/125 mL of pre-soaked groats
1/2 cup/125 mL of organic strawberries
2 tablespoons/30 mL of chopped pecans
1 teaspoon/5 mL of sucanat

Berry Good Morning Shake!
Single Serving

Blend all ingredients until smooth, pour into tall glass! Drink with gratitude!

In Blender add the following ingredients:

1 Tablespoon/15 mL of "Vega" Plant-Based Protein Powder
1 Tablespoon/15 mL of *Multi Greens Plus*
1 Tablespoon/15 mL of Ground Flax Seed
1/2 cup/125 mL of blueberries
1/2 cup/125 mL of strawberries
1/2 cup/125 mL of raspberries

SHAKE IT UP! Go Green Shake
Single Serving

Blend all ingredients until smooth, pour into tall glass! This hearty shake will hold you until Lunch! Green combination drinks are healing, stabilizing and calming, they have a relaxing centering effect as well as a boost to your immunities!

In Blender add the following ingredients:

1 tablespoon/15 mL of "Vega" Plant-Based Protein Powder
1 tablespoon/15 mL of *Multi Greens Plus*
1 tablespoon/15 mL of Ground Flax Seeds
1 teaspoon/5 mL of Spirulina
1 organic banana
1 Kiwi
1 slice of Pineapple
1 cup/250 mL of purified water

Breakfast Date Bread

Step One, In food processor add:
   2 cups/500 mL of soaked oat groats
   2 cups/500 mL of soaked buckwheat groats
   2 cups/500 mL of soaked barley
   2 cups/500 mL of Medjool dates (pitted) 1 cup/250 mL of raisins
   1 cup/250 mL of soaked walnuts
   1/2 cup/125 mL of almond flour
   1 cup/250 mL of ground flax seed
   1/2 cup/125 mL of purified water (filtered)
   1/4 cup/60 mL of maple syrup #2 (less refined)
   1/4 cup/60 mL of agave syrup
   1 tablespoon/15 mL of cinnamon

Process until dates and nuts are broken down into little pieces and the groats are more of a dough-like consistency! OR process less to give more texture! Add purified water a little at a time to get desired consistency and is easier to process and spread onto racks. For a fancier bread keep some nuts or fruit to chop small and fold into mixture before spreading onto Teflon coated racks.

Step Two, Dehydrate:

Spread this out onto 3 teflon coated racks and dehydrate 8-12 hours each side, at 110 degrees Fahrenheit, depending on how dry or how moist you like your bread. The first time I did it, I checked them at the 8 hour mark, turned them onto the rack peeling off the Teflon, returned them to the dehydrator for 10 more hours, so you see the flexibility is there! Top this with your favorite organic almond nut butter, banana and drizzle with raw honey and place a few pieces of seasonal fruit and enjoy!

This recipe will make 3 sheets cut into 9 pieces for a total of 27 pieces. Or 2 sheets of thicker, larger pieces, 24 hours one side, then 8 hours other side. Always monitor for desired level of moistness! Cut smaller if you like. Date Bread freezes well and is thawed and ready for Breakfast before you have made your

Greens Plus shake, literally it takes only a few minutes! You can warm up this delicious date bread by putting in dehydrator for an hour if you are serving brunch!

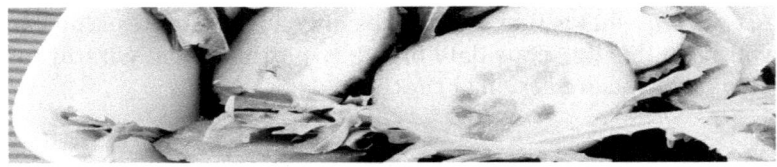

Lunches and Light Fare

Cabbage Slaw

Ingredients:

1/2 head of red/purple cabbage
1/2 head of green cabbage
2 carrots shredded
1/2 of diced yellow onion
1/4 cup/60 mL of sesame seeds

With sharp knife and cutting board chop vegetables into long pieces. Use mandolin if you prefer.

Dressing:

2 tablespoons/30 mL of hemp oil
2 tablespoons/30 mL of apple cider vinegar with mother
2 tablespoons/30 mL of pre-soaked cashews
1 tablespoon/15 mL of purified water
2 teaspoons/10 mL of sea salt
1 clove of garlic
Grinds of fresh black pepper

Blend with hand blender pour over Cabbage Slaw, toss and serve.

Spring Mix Salad

Toss with Raspberry Vinaigrette see recipe section. Place an edible flower on the side and serve!

Various fresh lettuce leaves:

  Dandelion greens
  Watercress
  Arugula
  Spinach
  Radicchio
  1/4 cup of sliced organic strawberries
  2 tablespoons/30 mL of slivered pre-soaked almonds
  2 tablespoons/30 mL of diced onion

Waldorf Salad
Single Serving

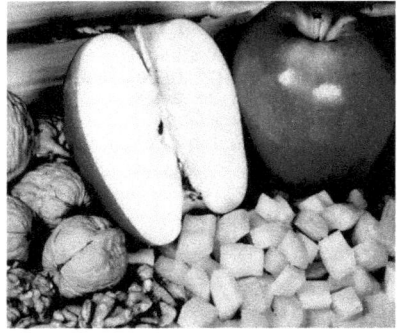

In large salad bowl add the following ingredients:

Rinsed fresh organic field greens and herbs
Half of a granny smith or Cortland apple cut into wedges
6 chopped pre-soaked walnuts
1/2 stalk of finely sliced organic celery

Top with a Vinaigrette salad dressing.

*Tip Dip apple slices in lemon juice so apple does not turn brown.

Spinach Salad

Ingredients:

2 cups/500 mL of baby spinach leaves
4 crimini mushrooms chopped
2 tablespoons/30 mL of chopped onion
1 mandarin orange, divided into sections
1 tablespoon/15 mL of pre-soaked sunflower seeds
6 olives

Toss with Olive Oil Vinaigrette:

1 tablespoon/15 mL of cold pressed extra virgin olive oil
1 tablespoon/15 mL of apple cider vinegar with mother
1 teaspoon/5 mL of sea salt
grinds of fresh ground pepper

Always rinse fresh produce from supermarket before storing in fridge.

THIN-CRUST-ZAA Thin Crust Veggie Pizza

Tomato Paste - In Blender add the following ingredients:

1 cup/250 mL of dry sun-dried tomatoes
1/2 cup/125 mL of olive oil
1/2 cup/125 mL of Nama Shoyu
1/4 cup/60 mL of Braggs soy flavouring
1/4 cup/60 mL of Apple Cider Vinegar with Mother
1/4 fresh squeezed lemon
4 cloves of garlic
2 tablespoons/30 mL of chopped oregano
2 tablespoons/30 mL of chopped cilantro
1 teaspoon/5 mL of sea salt

Process until paste like texture with all ingredients totally processed into spreadable texture. Set aside.

Nut Cheese - In Food Processor add the following ingredients:
>1 cup/250 mL of pre-soaked sunflower seeds
>Juice of one lemon
>2 cloves of garlic
>1 teaspoon/5 mL of sea salt

Water to get desired consistency, introduce water slowly then blend, add little at a time until satisfied. Set aside.

Assembly:
Spread Tomato paste on Herbed Onion Bread shaped in Triangles; see recipe section. Top with your choice of sliced vegetables such as olives, mushrooms, green and yellow peppers. Top sliced vegetables with Nut Cheese.

- If you wish, Warm in dehydrator at 105 degrees Fahrenheit for half an hour, enjoy!

Greek Pizza

Enough for 8-16, depending how thick you spread this yummy spread!

For this recipe, you will use the Savoury Herb Onion Bread as a base.

Greek Pizza Spread - In Food Processor Add:
>2 cups/500 mL pre-soaked cashews
>2 cups/500 mL soaked chick peas
>1/2 cup/125 mL of lemon juice
>1/4 cup/60 mL Tahini Sauce
>1/4 cup/60 mL of water (you may need more for desired consistency)
>1 tablespoon/15 mL of olive oil
>2 cloves of garlic
>1/2 teaspoon/2 mL of cumin

Blend until smooth, spread as thickly as desired onto Savoury Herb Onion Bread.

Toppings:
>Organic spinach, lettuces, herbs chopped up small
>Diced onions finely chopped
>Red peppers finely chopped

Sundried tomatoes chopped in tiny pieces
Cherry tomatoes halved
Olives, your favourite type cut in half
Cucumber, sliced & cut into wedges
Sprouted mung beans

Enjoy! Nothing says Friday like pizza!

Corny Chowder

Blend at high speed in Vita Mix until steam comes out of lid, pour into bowls, store remaining in fridge, will keep a few days, freeze if desired to keep longer. Enjoy!

In Blender add the following ingredients:

6 cups/1.5 L of fresh corn niblets
2 1/2 cups/750 mL of water
1/2 cup/125 mL of pre-soaked macadamia nuts
2 teaspoons/10 mL of sea salt
1/2 teaspoon/2 mL of cayenne pepper

BEANIE BABYYY! 100% Raw Sprouted Bean Salad
In medium bowl add the following ingredients:

1 cup of your choice of sprouted beans
1 red diced pepper
1 green diced pepper
1 yellow diced pepper
1/2 organic cucumber quartered and sliced
1 cup/250 mL of diced celery
1/2 sweet onion diced
1 cup/250 mL of cherry tomatoes halved
1 tablespoon/15 mL of hemp seeds
2 jalapeno peppers chopped into little rings (optional for added heat)

Vinaigrette dressing:

    3 tablespoons/45 mL of hemp oil
    3 tablespoons/45 mL of apple cider vinegar with mother
    2 cloves of garlic minced
    1/2 cup/125 mL of a sweet onion diced
    2 teaspoons/10 mL of sea salt

LIMEY SOUP Curry Carrot Soup

In Vita Mix Blender blend all ingredients at high for 2 minutes, you will see steam in a Vita Mix blender, but it will not heat above 120 degrees F.

- This soup goes well accompanied by a Waldorf Salad!

In Vita Mix Blender add the following ingredients:

    Juice of 6 carrots
    1/2 stalk of celery
    1/2 a medium onion
    1/2 cup/125 mL of macadamia nuts
    1/3 cup/100 mL of coconut meat
    Squeezed juice from 1/2 lime
    1 teaspoon/5 mL of curry paste
    1/2 tsp/2 mL of lime zest to garnish

Autumn Stew

Blend to point of steam coming from lid. These blenders are perfect for heating up ingredients to a safe temperature and not killing the nutrients. Place in large bowl, set aside.
In Vita Mix Blender add all the following ingredients:

    1 tomato
    1 sweet red pepper
    1/2 of large cucumber
    1 habenaro chili pepper
    1 clove of garlic
    1/4 of large sweet onion
    1/2 cup/125 mL of olive oil
    Add sea salt to taste!

Optional, if you prefer a thick base, add one can of chick peas or mixed beans at this stage as a thickener.

Process ingredients to point of steam coming from lid.

In Vita Mix Blender add the following ingredients:
    2 cups/500 mL of Organic Vegetable Broth
    1 1/2 cups/375 mL of coconut milk
    2 tablespoons/30 mL of curry paste

Mix with gazpacho base stored in large bowl, mix well, add sea salt to taste! Pour into soup bowls to serve, decorate with cilantro leaves.

Final Step. Add the following ingredients to the above listed ingredients in the Vita Mix last, but only pulse/process, for a second, don't puree. You want texture in your soup so you have something to chew.

    1 can/14 fl oz./398 mL of organic chick peas
    1/2 green pepper
    1/2 red pepper

SKINNY STICKS Veggie Nofries

Assembly:

Peel avocado, removing seed and slice avocado into thin wedges. Cut small sweet potato leaving skin intact, into French fry shapes. Cut zucchini, leaving skin intact into French fry shapes discarding centre row of seeds. When all vegetables are cut into desired shapes take the zucchini and sweet potato and coat in the olive oil and set aside. Mix the spice coating ingredients until evenly blended, place in bowl. Roll each vegetable in below blended spice mixture using a fork and place on teflon coated dehydrator rack, do not over crowd. Dehydrate for 1 hour. Enjoy with your favourite salad or perhaps it will be a fun finger food night with salsa, or my personal favourite our ketchup! Whatever the occasion Enjoy!

Ingredients:

    1 organic avocado
    1 small organic sweet potato
    1 organic medium zucchini

Spice Coating Ingredients:

    1/2 cup/125 mL of ground flax seeds
    1 tablespoon/15 mL of nutritional yeast
    2 teaspoons/10 mL of chili powder
    2 teaspoons/10 mL of dried minced garlic (good for added crunch)
    2 teaspoons/10 mL of cumin
    2 teaspoons/10 mL of garam masala
    2 teaspoons/10 mL of Sea Salt

- Extra virgin cold-pressed olive oil, to coat zucchini and sweet potato before rolling into spice coating

Living the Raw Live Vegan Lifestyle

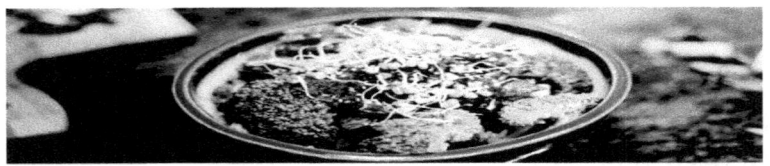

Main Meals

Thai Curry, "RLV" Style!
Curry Sauce - Put following ingredients in blender:
1 cup/250 mL of coconut milk
2 medium size organic vine ripened tomatoes
1 medium/large organic avocado
1 bunch of organic cilantro
1/2 cup /125 mL of yellow onion
1/2 cup/125 mL of raw coconut flakes
1 tablespoon/15 mL of fresh ginger
1 clove of garlic
1 tablespoon/15 mL of curry powder
1 tablespoon/15 mL of lemon juice
1 tablespoon/15 mL of Nama Shoyu
2 Madjool dates

Process all of the above ingredients until creamy sauce like consistency. Season with sea salt and pepper to taste!

For Rice - In food processor pulse to rice size consistency
1 head of cauliflower chopped

In colander:
1 bunch of baby bok choy leaves that have been wilted with 120 degree F. water left to sit in strainer until ready to assemble.

Garnish ingredients:
Sweet red pepper cut into thin strips
Fresh mung bean sprouts
Shredded organic carrots
1 tablespoon/15 mL of shredded organic raw cashews chopped or whole per serving

Assembly:
On plates assemble bok choy leaves onto center of plate, top with 1 cup/250 mL of cauliflower rice, drizzle curry sauce over the rice, top with garnish and again a little more curry sauce. Serve to eager recipients and enjoy!

Asian Stir, Not Fry

Step One: Rice Like Base - In food processor add:
Organic cauliflower

This will process cauliflower down to small rice-size pieces. Set aside.

Step Two: Designer Cut Vegetables:
Cut up vegetables in interesting shapes, simulating Chinese food. Cut carrots into match stick shapes, the peppers into long strips, shred the cabbage, chunk the pineapple, leave the snow peas whole, and cut the broccoli into florettes.

Step Three: Heat to Warm
Vegetables can then be placed into a colander and set in sink. Heat kettle to almost a boil, let cook and pour water over vegetables. This will give them the look of being steamed, but they are not, as the water runs through the colander. It doesn't cook the vegetables, but it definitely warms and softens them! Set aside.

Step Four: The Sauce
In Vita Mix Blender add:
1/2 cup/125 mL of nama shoyu
1/2 cup/125 mL of apple cider Vinegar with Mother
1/4 cup/60 mL water
1/4 cup/60 mL of olive oil
1/4 cup/60 mL dried tomatoes
1/4 cup/60 mL dates
2 Tablespoons/30 mL of agave syrup
2 Teaspoons/10 mL of dry mustard
1 Teaspoon/5mL of fresh grated ginger
2 cloves of garlic
Juice of one Lemon
Sea Salt to taste, must taste prior to adding!

Step Five: Final topping
Top with 1/2 cup/125 mL of pre-soaked cashews, 1/2 cup/125 mL of pre-soaked almonds, fresh mung bean sprouts, Arame seaweed, chunked pineapple (1/2 of fresh whole pineapple),and sesame seeds. Set aside to put on top right before serving!

Step Six: The Assembly, A Work of Art!
Place rice-like base on the bottom of a serving dish. Top with fresh, almost steamed vegetables. Then top with the sauce that was blended to the point of heating up. Last, but not least, add topping of nuts, seeds, beans, pineapple, arame and sprouts!

Mock Turkey Roll

Always have a little purified water available to mix into the above, in case the mixture is too dry. This makes it easier to shape. Shape it into a roll, or into patties, OR into a Turkey! Place on a teflon coated rack. Dehydrate for 4 - 6 hours at 118 degrees Fahrenheit. Decorate the roll with a hint of paprika and parsley. I serve it with broccoli, carrots, and cauliflower. Place veggies in a colander, and pour hot water over them, to give them a darker colour and warmth, before serving. Dried cranberries can be rehydrated with orange juice, add a date, run through processor and serve! I top my Mock Turkey Roll with Portobello Mushroom Gravy. Check out the recipe section on Dressings, Sauces and Condiments!

In Food Processor add the following ingredients:

2 cups/500 mL of celery
2 cups/500 mL of shitake mushrooms
1 cup/250 mL of soaked almonds
1 cup/250 mL of soaked walnuts
1 cup/250 mL of sunflower seeds
1 cup/250 mL of cashews
1 cup/250 mL of onion
1 cup/250 mL of carrot
1 cup/250 mL of dried cranberries
1 cup/250 mL of ground flax
3/4 cup/180 ml of hemp oil
1/4 cup/60 mL of hemp seed
1 tablespoon/15 mL of parsley
1 tablespoon/15 mL of paprika
1 tablespoon/15 mL of savory
1 tablespoon/15 mL of cumin
1 tablespoon/15 mL of garam marsala
1 tablespoon/15 mL of pepper
1 tablespoon/15 mL of sea salt

Sea Kelp Helps! Sea Noodle Salad

This serves two, with leftovers for a lucky one.

This is a wonderfully easy and bountiful dish from the SEA!!

Assembly:

Mix dressing ingredients well by hand or use tall cylinder container with hand blender to blend into puree consistency. Portion out individual bowls of sea kelp noodles, top with assorted veggies, drizzle delicious dressing over top of your veggies and noodles. Top with broccoli and radish sprouts. Impress your guests and palate by adding a dash of black sesame seeds!

In a bowl add the following ingredients:

2 packages Sea Kelp noodles, rinse and separate the kelp strands.
1 large carrot. I like to peel mine into thin slices.
10 green pea pods, diced.
1/2 red pepper, thinly sliced.
1/2 orange pepper, thinly sliced.
1/2 yellow pepper, thinly sliced.
broccoli and radish sprouts.

Dressing - In a bowl add:

1/2 clove minced garlic.
1 tablespoon/15 mL minced ginger.
1/2 cup/125 mL safflower oil.
1/4 cup/60 mL lemon juice.
2 tablespoons/30 mL tahini.
1 teaspoon/5 mL light miso.
dash of sea salt.

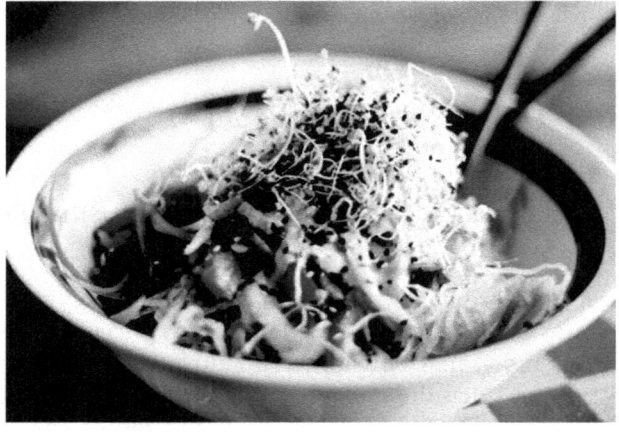

Green Party Kale and Broccoli with Tahini Sauce

Assembly:

In Large Colander add cut up Kale leaves, stem removed, cut up broccoli heads and stems, all in small bite size pieces. Set Colander in sink and rinse with water, leave to drain.

Take a kettle of hot water, not boiling, 120 degrees F., and pour over kale/broccoli mixture in colander and allow hot water to pour through, place this warmed mix into individual serving bowls, top with assortment of vegetables and walnuts, pour on the Tahini sauce, toss until everything is well coated. Top with sprouted mung beans.

Ingredients - Wash and set aside:

Large bunch of organic kale
1/4 of organic yellow onion diced fine
1/4 cup/60 mL of kernels from organic corn
4 organic crimini mushrooms diced fine sprouted mung beans
8 large pre-soaked walnuts chopped into small pieces.

"Tahini Sauce" - In Blender add:

Juice from 1 orange
1/2 teaspoon/2 mL of sesame oil
1 1/2/25 mL tablespoons of tahini paste
2 tablespoons/30 mL of cold pressed olive oil
2 tablespoons/30 mL of white balsamic vinegar
1 tablespoon/15 mL of miso

Blend and set aside.

ON TOP OF OLD SMOKEY
Rawghetti & Mock Meat Balls

Tomato Sauce - In Blender add the following ingredients:
4 organic vine-ripened tomatoes
2 Red Peppers
4 tablespoons/60 mL of sun-dried tomato powder OR (12 sun-dried tomatoes)
1/4 onion
3 cloves of garlic
2 dates
2 tablespoons/30 mL of olive oil
2 tablespoons/30 mL of diced basil leaves OR (1 tablespoon/15 mL of dried basil)
2 tablespoons/30 mL of diced fresh oregano OR (1 tablespoon/15 mL of dried oregano)
dried chili peppers (add one at a time and taste for desired heat)
1 teaspoon/5 mL of sea salt

For a thicker sauce slice your tomatoes and drain the liquid and remove the seeds, using only the meat and skin of the tomato, plus you could add more sun-dried tomatoes to get the desired thickness, this would give you a wonderful Marinara, add more liquid and another vegetable, perhaps zucchini and get an antipesto! You are as limited as your creativity! If you crave salt add yeast flakes, Braggs, miso or sea-salt inter-changeably to get the desired salty taste.

Place tomato sauce in pie plate or any casserole dish and place in dehydrator at 118 degrees Fahrenheit and warm up for about 3 hours.

Noodles:

3 organic zucchinis medium sized or 2 large. Use a peeler, specially designed to grate vegetable into long noodle like thin strips. Do not grate zucchini into the seeded core, use only the outer layer toward the centre core. Set aside.

Cheesy-Taste Topping - In Blender add the following ingredients:
- 2 cups/500 mL of soaked nuts of choice, this can be cashews, macadamia, sunflower seeds, brazil nuts or a combination of all of these! You do not have to dry them if they are presently stored in refrigerator as you will be adding water to them!
- 3 cloves of garlic
- 1 teaspoon/5 mL of nutritional yeast flakes
- 1 teaspoon/5mL of Himalayan Sea Salt
- 1/2 cup/125 mL of water, ***add a little at a time and continue to blend you may need less or more depending on desired consistency.

Mock Meatballs:

See Savoury Herb Onion Bread Recipe; we use this recipe to shape into meatballs!

Assembly:

On dinner plates distribute evenly zucchini noodles, separating the noodles with a fork. Pour Tomato Sauce over top of zucchini noodles. Place Mock Meatballs over top of tomato sauce. Dab "nut cheese" on top of "Mock Spaghetti and Meatballs."

TIP Another option in preparation of this dish is if you are in a hurry and have a Vita Mix Blender you can blend tomato sauce until steam appears through the lid, pour this over the noodles add the mock meatballs, top with mock cheese serve and enjoy!

BROC RAWKS RED CABBAGE-N-BROCCOLI

Serving for 2

In colander add first 4 ingredients. Pour hot water (no more than 118 degrees Fahrenheit over the vegetables. Colors will be vibrant! Place in large Bowl.

For Sauce add last 5 ingredients to blender and puree. Pour sauce over vegetables in large bowl to coat. Top with sprouts!

Ingredients:

1/4 head of red cabbage chopped
2 cups/500 ml of broccoli florettes
1/4 cup/60 ml of sunflower seeds
2 carrots finely sliced (optional)
1/4 cup/60 ml hempseed oil
1/4 cup/60 ml cold-pressed virgin olive oil
2 Umeboshi plums pickled.
Sea salt and ground black pepper to taste.

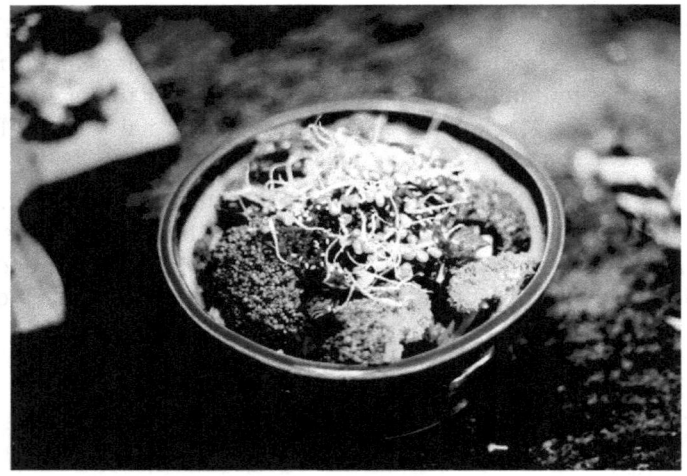

IN A HURRY CURRY Curry Sea Noodles

Noodles:

> 1 package of sea kelp noodles
> Ingredients for Curry Sauce
> 1 cup/250 mL of water
> 1/2 cup/125 mL of Macadamia nuts
> 1/4 cup/60 mL of coconut meat
> 1 tablespoon/15 mL curry paste
> 2 teaspoons/10 mL of chili paste
> 1/2 teaspoon/2 mL of sea salt

Assembly:

Rinse sea kelp noodles and leave in colander to drain. In Blender blend all ingredients for curry sauce until thick rich creamy texture, taste to test for desired flavour. Divide sea kelp noodles into two bowls. Top noodles with the following ingredients, divide evenly.

> Shave 1/4 cup/60 mL kernels of corn from cob
> 1/2 cup/125 mL Bell Peppers diced: red, green, orange
> 1/4 cup/60 mL celery diced

Pour Rich creamy curry sauce on top and add a dash of cayenne pepper on top. Enjoy!

Sushi Mooshi Nori Rolls

Assembly:

Spread olive tapenade in narrow row down narrow end of nori roll. Lay thin slivers of vegetables down the centre on top of the tapenade, leave some colourful vegetable sticks sticking out at each end, these will provide decorative nori rolls in the centre of your display dish. Wrap tightly rolling over empty section of sheet toward end, when you get to last inch of empty nori sheet, dip finger in rice wine vinegar, rub lightly end of nori sheet and complete the roll, leaving the weight of the roll to seal the edge. I cut each end of the nori roll longer than the ones in the middle so that they do stand out in the centre of the display dish! Serve with small serving dish of wasabi paste and small serving dish of Nama Shoyu. Enjoy!

Olive Tapenade filling - In food processor add ingredients:

1 cup/250 mL of olives
1 cup/250 mL of pre-soaked sunflower seeds
2 Tablespoons/30 mL of minced garlic
2 Tablespoons/30 mL of minced scallions
2 Tablespoons/30 mL of Old Style Mustard
2 Tablespoons/30 mL of Olive Oil
2 Tablespoons/30 mL of Nama Shyu
2 Tablespoons/30 mL of fresh minced dill
2 Tablespoons/30 mL of fresh minced cilantro

Process above ingredients until paste like consistency, set mixture aside.

Slice the following vegetables into long match stick slivers:

red pepper
carrot
cucumber
avocado

Set slivered vegetables aside.

In small finger bowl have 1 tablespoon/15 mL of rice wine vinegar to seal outer edge of nori roll, set aside.

NUTTY BUGGERS Veggie Nut Burgers

In Food Processor add the following ingredients:

2 cups/500 mL of raw pre-soaked almonds
2 cups/500 mL of raw pre-soaked sunflower seeds
2 cups/500 mL of raw pre-soaked walnuts
2 cups/500 mL of pre-soaked ground flax seed

* TIP Pre-soaked nuts do not have to be dried as we will be adding liquid to them.

Pulse to chop stage, place chopped nuts in large bowl.

In Food Processor add the following ingredients:

3 cups/750 mL of mushrooms
1 yellow onion
2 cups/500 mL of chopped celery
3 carrots
1 red pepper
1 zucchini

Process to fine chop stage, place in large bowl with nuts, set aside.

On cutting board with sharp knife, finely chop the following ingredients:

Cloves of 1 garlic bulb finely chopped
1/2 bunch of parsley leaves chopped fine
1/2 bunch of tarragon leaves chopped fine
1/2 bunch of cilantro leaves chopped fine

Add finely chopped herbs and garlic to large bowl of processed nuts.

In small bowl add the following liquids:

1/2 cup/125 mL of Flax oil
1 1/2/375 mL cup of Nama Shoyu
1/2 cup/125 mL of Braggs Liquid Soy, all purpose flavouring

Mix above liquids with hand blender and add to large bowl of dry ingredients.

Assembly:

Mix large batch well, taste to see if anything is missing, then spoon onto teflon coated racks and shape into patties or small round balls for mock meat balls, (great for dipping!). Dehydrate at 105 degrees Fahrenheit for 12 hours one side and then remove from teflon coated rack and flip on wire rack without teflon and continue to dehydrate for another 12-18 hours depending on how dry you want them to be. What I like about this recipe is that they are savoury, you can grab and go knowing you have your protein, veggies and high quality fibre, all in one! Enjoy Nut Burger on Herbed Onion Bread with mustard or as

Mock Meat Balls in Marinara Sauce on your favourite veggie noodles!

CHICKEN LITTLE A Little Like Chicken

Process ingredients to fine chop stage, add water as needed for desired texture, process lightly with short bursts of power. Served on a romaine leaf, scoop onto romaine leaf, top with fine chopped red, green, yellow peppers. (Add spices to suit your palate, you know what you like in a "chicken-taste" sandwich it could be chili peppers! Have fun!) Add a side order of broccoli and baby carrots! On the raw live vegan plan it is okay to chop up into small pieces broccoli and carrots and place in colander in sink and pour *almost boiling water* over, the water will run off and not cook the vegetables. I bring kettle to boil and let temperature cool down close to 120 degrees F. Enjoy a leafy green vegetable salad add a few mandarin orange slices and some radish sprouts to a bowl of baby greens, top with a raspberry vinaigrette.

In food processor add the following ingredients:

1/4 cup/60 mL of soaked sunflower seeds,
1/4 cup/60 mL of soaked almonds,
1/4 cup/60 mL of celery ,
1/4 cup/60 mL of white onion,
1 tablespoon/15 mL of fresh squeezed lemon,
1 tablespoon/15 mL of fresh summer savory,
1 teaspoom/5 mL of sea salt.
1/4 teaspoon/1 mL of paprika,
1/2 teaspoon/2 mL of light miso,

YUMMY YAKI
Teriyaki Vegetables With Pineapple Marinade

Step One

In Juicer put half of a cored and trimmed pineapple, enough to yield a 1/4 cup/60 mL of juice, pour into food processor and then add:

- 1 tablespoon/15 mL of tamari
- 2 teaspoons/10 mL of agave syrup
- 2 teaspoons/10 mL sesame oil
- 2 teaspoons/10 mL of squeezed lemon juice
- 1 teaspoon of olive oil
- 1 teaspoon/5 mL of mustard powder
- 1 teaspoon/5 mL of nama shoyu
- 1 teaspoon/5 mL of chopped fine onion
- 1 clove of fine chopped garlic
- 1 teaspoon/5 mL of sesame seeds
- 1/4 teaspoon 1 mL of grated ginger
- Dash of cayenne pepper.

Process to puree consistency.

Step Two

Place marinade in dehydrator at 115 degrees F., for 1 hour to reduce. Right before serving, rinse your choice of fresh vegetables. I use bok choy, broccoli, mushrooms, peppers, carrots, chop and place in colander in sink. Pour *almost boiling water* over vegetables in colander, slowly allowing the water to wash the vegetables and drain into the sink, this is not like placing vegetables into boiling water long enough to kill the enzymes, in fact I bring kettle to boil then let cool to 120 degrees F. The vegetables will be colorful and crisp, arrange on plates, pour marinade over them. Top with 1/4 cup/60 mL of fresh pineapple sliced in chunks and 2 tablespoons/30 mL of cashews, and of course some sprouts of your choice. Try chop sticks for fun, you certainly will be concentrating on the food you are eating by using these implements!

Mockfish Stuffed Red Peppers
"ANOTHER FISH FAKE"

In a food processor add the following ingredients:

1/4 cup/60 mL of soaked and dried sunflower seeds
1/4 cup/60 mL of soaked and dried almonds
1/4 cup/60 mL of celery
1/4 cup/60 mL of Spanish onion
2 tablespoon/30 mL fresh cilantro
2 tablespoon/30 mL fresh dill
1 clove of garlic
1 tablespoon/15 mL of micro-planed carrot
1 tablespoon/15 mL of dried arame (seaweed)
1 tablespoon/15 mL of fresh squeezed lime juice
1 teaspoon/5 mL of fresh chopped dill
1/2 teaspoon/2 mL of miso

This mockfish is much yummier then the actual tuna!! In my humble opinion.

Process to chunk like consistency, scoop 1/2 cup into your halved red peppers.

QUI RAWWWW
"Quinoa Salad" Raw Live Vegan Style

Blend with hand blender dressing until all ingredients pureed. Pour dressing over vegetable mix and toss to cover. On each plate place 1/2 cup/125 mL of bean sprouts, then 1 cup of the vegetable mix, top with 1/4 cup of freshly sprouted quinoa. Congratulations you are about to enjoy the 100% *raw* version of the quinoa salad!

In large bowl put:

1 cup/250 mL of chopped green peppers
1 cup/250mL yellow peppers
1 cup/250 mL red peppers

1 cup/250 mL of chopped cucumber
1 cup/250 mL of fine chopped celery
1 cup/250 mL of halved cherry tomatoes
1/2 cup/125 mL of finely shredded carrots
1/4 cup/60 mL of assorted raw seeds (sesame, sunflower, pumpkin)
1/2 cup125 mL of chopped onion
1/2 cup/125 mL of sliced radishes
1/4 cup/60 mL of dried unsweetened cranberries
3 jalapeno peppers thinly chopped into rings
1/4 cup/60 mL of fresh sprouted quinoa seeds

Dressing: In bowl add the following ingredients:

1/4 cup/60 mL of olive oil
1/4 cup/60 mL of apple cider vinegar with mother
1 clove of garlic minced
1 sprig of parsley finely chopped
1 sprig of oregano finely chopped
1 sprig of cilantro finely chopped

Soft Shell Corn Tortillas

In Blender add the following ingredients:

4 cups/1000 mL of organic yellow peppers
3 cups/750 mL of fresh organic corn nibs straight off the cob
1 cup/250 mL of fresh organic zucchini, peeled & chopped
1 organic avocado, peeled, pit removed
3 tablespoons/45 mL of psyllium powder
1 tablespoon/15 mL of nutritional yeast flakes
1 tablespoon/15 mL of organic lime or lemon juice freshly squeezed

Blend until smooth, using plunger to get thorough blend of all ingredients. The psyllium not only adds quality fibre but gives the tortilla shell its' elasticity. Work fast as this mix thickens rapidly. With 1/2 cup measure you should be able to measure out 8 tortilla shells. Place mixture from 1/2 cup measure onto teflon coated dehydrator racks and dehydrate for 4 hours at 105 degrees Fahrenheit. Then flip tortillas off the teflon sheet onto wire racks and continue to dehydrate for 1 1/2 to 2 hours.

A good base for tortillas is guacamole.

Guacamole - In bowl add the following ingredients:

1 organic avocado, peeled and pit removed
1 clove of organic garlic diced fine
juice from 1/2 of fresh organic lime or lemon
dash of sea salt and pepper, to taste (optional)

Toppings for Tortilla:

kale leaves
guacamole
chopped red pepper
corn niblets
fresh sprouted mung beans

Preparation:

Top each tortilla with a kale leaf. Place some guacamole mix on top of kale leaf. Top with red pepper pieces. Top with corn niblets. Top with fresh sprouted mung beans. Enjoy, make extra for impromptu guests!

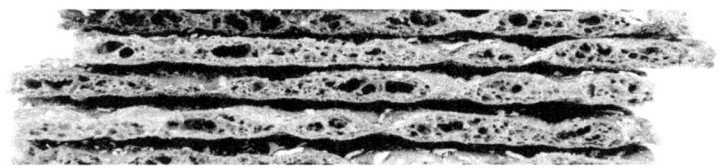

Breads & Crackers

Fire Crackers

Step One, In a mixing bowl add the following ingredients:

   4 cups/1 L pre-soaked flax seeds that have soaked for 6-8 hours.
   4 cups/1 L ground flax flour.
Set ingredients aside.

Step Two, In a food processor add the following ingredients:

   3 large tomatoes
   1 red pepper
   1/2 cup/125 mL of chopped fine mixed hot peppers - habanero, cherry, chili, etc.
   2 tablespoons/30 mL. sea salt
   1/2 cup/125 mL corn
   1 onion
   4 cloves garlic
   1 cup/250 mL of water (optional, add what you need, add hot sauce/chilies to make it hotter)

Process vegetables to fine chop stage. Add the processed chopped vegetables to the bowl of ground flax and flax seeds. Mix thoroughly, gradually adding the water as you mix it into a thick, yet spreadable mixture.

Step Three, Dehydrate

Place 2 cups/500 mL of thoroughly mixed mixture on teflon-lined dehydrator rack, spread roughly, corner to corner. To get a perfect level of thickness, take a second teflon sheet, place on top of roughly spread mixture and then with rolling pin roll out corner to corner, when you remove the teflon sheet off the top you can trim sides to make a perfect square and then you can cut strips, running a dull knife horizontally and vertically to create the size of crackers you would like. Place racks in dehydrator at 118 degrees Fahrenheit for 10-12 hours and then take out of dehydrator, flip over, remove teflon sheet, return to dehydrator for 10-12 hours more at 118 degrees Fahrenheit or more for desired crispness!

This recipe makes 4 racks of crackers. They will store easily for a month, if they last that long!

Enjoy!

Veggie Crackers

Step One, In a large bowl add the following ingredients:

3 cups/750 mL pre-soaked Flax seeds
2 cups/500 mL Flax powder (add more if necessary)

Step Two, In Food Processor add the following ingredients:

6 sun-dried tomatoes
1 large sweet red pepper
4 whole tomatoes
1 zucchini
3 cloves of garlic
1 sweet white onion
1/4 cup/60 mL of fresh cilantro
1 tablespoon/15 mL of sea salt
1 tablespoon/15 mL of sucanat
4 sweet peppers *I am replacing the chili peppers with these, because I came up with a knock your socks off spicy cracker recipe which is under FIRE CRACKERS! These ones will turn out just veggieriffic!

Add the above vegetable mixture to large bowl of pre-soaked flax seed and ground flax flour mixture, fold in until all ingredients are well blended.

Step Three, Dehydrate

The mixture should be stiff and heavy. If it is too soupy add more flax flour; the thickness is your choice. Spread out onto teflon lined dehydrator racks. Do not be afraid to spread thinly.

Remember, the thicker it is, the longer it will take to dehydrate. Dehydrate at 110 degrees Fahrenheit for 12 hours, then flip onto rack. Remove teflon and dehydrate for 12 hours more. If crackers are very thick or very moist, continue to dehydrate longer.

Score your crackers in any shape you like. Adjust this recipe to suit your taste, this is what it's all about! This recipe makes 4 racks of crackers. They store easily for one month, but keep an eye on them, they will disappear!

JUNGIAN BREAD Savoury Herb Onion Bread

Step One, In Large Bowl add:

2 cups/500 mL of ground Flax Seed

Step Two, In Dry Blender container of Vita Mix add:

2 cups/500 mL of ground sunflower seeds (pre-soaked and dried)
Process until flour like consistency.

Step Three, Mandolin

3 Large Onions sliced thin!

Step Four, In Food Processor add the following ingredients:

Chunks of onion that did not slice small or half of another onion,
1 cup/250 mL of Namo Shoyu
1/2 cup/125 mL of Hemp oil
1/4 cup/60 mL Braggs Soy Flavouring
Juice of 1 Lemon
1 tablespoon/15 mL of Oregano
1 tablespoon/15 mL of Thyme
1 tablespoon/15 mL of Italian Seasoning
Garlic clove/powder to taste, (optional)
1 tablespoon/15 mL of Fresh dill (optional)

Process liquids and spices, pour liquid over large bowl of dry ingredients and onions, fold ingredients over, continually, until well mixed, if too difficult and batter too stiff, add a little water. Also keep in mind, you can add twice the amount of dry and liquid measures to the same original amount of onions to get a thicker bread.

Step Five, Dehydrate

Spread bread dough out onto teflon-lined dehydrator racks. Score into desired shapes, triangles or squares for pizzas or rectangular for soup. For Mock Meat Balls, process remaining batter and onions to form smooth dough, use a teaspoon to drop dough balls onto teflon lined dehydrator racks. If you like the consistency of the dough used for mock meatballs you can process whole batch and roll out bread that way too! Dehydrate 12 hours on one side, flip, remove teflon sheet, return to dehydrate 12 hours more on the other side. The mock meatballs, require only 6 hours on one side, roll off teflon sheet place onto rack and return to dehydrate 6 hours more, you decide how dry you prefer, finished product.

This will make 3 racks of bread, 27 pieces, or 2 racks of bread, and one rack of mock meatballs!

- This bread is a staple in our diet now, and I admittedly dream about it sometimes, hence it's name- Jungian Bread!

Enjoy!

Sea-Biscuits

Step One, In the a food processor add the following ingredients:

- 4 cups/1 L of pre-soaked flax seeds, seeds that have soaked 6-8 hours.
- 4 cups/1 L ground flax.
- 1 sweet onion chopped
- 6 stalks celery
- 4 cloves garlic
- 1/4 cup/60 mL dill
- 2 tablespoons/30 mL of nama shoyu

Process vegetables and chop to fine chop stage then set aside in large bowl:

Step Two, In Dry Blender of Vita Mix add the following ingredients:

> 1/4 cup/60 mL dulce - diced.
> 1/4 cup/60 mL dried kelp - mine comes in sheets; I use my food scissors to cut it.

The dulce and dried kelp should be finely chopped. If you do not have a Vita Mix with the dry ingredients blender attachment, just take a little extra time and break up both the dulce and the kelp into small flecks by taking a chef knife and place the blade in a rocking motion over the sea kelp and rock forward and backward chopping the dulse and kelp into fine bits. Add dry chopped bits/powder sea product to large bowl of chopped vegetables and flax.

Step Three, mix thoroughly!

Add what you need from approximately 1 1/2 cups of water gradually as you mix it into a thick yet spreadable mixture. I always have a cup and 1/2 of water on hand to add to mixture so that the mix is spreadable.

Step Four, Dehydrator

Take a teflon-lined dehydrator rack and place 2 cups of mixture onto sheet and spread evenly, this is accomplished easily by using a second teflon sheet and a rolling pin, rolling pin never comes in contact with mix as it is separated by second sheet of teflon, this will give you an even height for equal dehydration. The best part is, after you remove the top teflon sheet after rolling mixture out you can now trim sides to make a perfect square, you can patch too, this type of food prep is very forgiving! Make crackers whatever shape and size that appeals to you, if you had time and the cracker was for company to go with a soup little fish cookie cutters would be over the top for presentation! Place in Dehydrator at 118 degrees F., for 10-12 hours, then turn over, remove teflon sheet and place back in dehydrator for 10-12 hours more for desired crispness. This recipe makes 4 racks of crackers. They will store easily for a month! Enjoy!

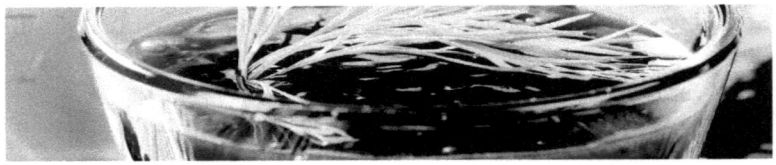

Dips & Spreads

Tzatsiki

Place the above ingredients in a food processor, process until creamy like consistency.
In Food Processor add:

- 1 cucumber, peeled
- 2 cloves of garlic
- 1 avocado,
- Peeled, pit removed
- 2 tablespoons/30 mL of olive oil
- 1 teaspoon/5 mL of sea salt
- 1 teaspoon/5 mL of dried mint

Olive Tapenade

Blend in a food processor until chunky consistency, then serve.
In Food Processor add:

- 1 cup/250 mL of mixed olives
- 1 clove of garlic minced
- 2 fresh basil leaves
- 1 tablespoon/15 mL of fresh squeezed lemon juice
- 2 tablespoons/30 mL of extra virgin olive oil
- 2 tablespoons/30 mL of capers

Spinach Dip

Depending if you want the spinach visible, you can leave it in a bowl chopped fine, then in blender blend the rest of the ingredients and mix with chopped spinach, chill in fridge until ready to serve.

In Food Processor add:

   10 oz of organic spinach chopped
   1/2 of Spanish onion
   1 ½ cup/375 mL cashews, soaked and dehydrated
   1 cup/250 mL of purified water
   1/2 cup/125 mL lemon juice
   2 tablespoons/30 mL of nutritional flakes
   4 cloves garlic
   2 teaspoons/10 mL of sea salt
   1 teaspoon/5 mL of psyllium husk

Guacamole

Place the above ingredients in a food processor, process until creamy like consistency.

In Food Processor add:

   2 avocados, peeled and pit removed
   1/2 small onion
   juice from one fresh lemon
   2 cloves of garlic
   1/2 jalapeno pepper
   1 teaspoon/5 mL of ground cumin
   1 teaspoon/5 mL of sea salt

Onion Cheez

Process in food processor adding enough water slowly for desired consistency.

In Food Processor add:

2 cups/500 mL of pre-soaked almonds
2 tablespoons/30 mL of light miso
3 tablespoons/45 mL of chopped green onion
2 teaspoons/10 mL of sea salt
Water, add as needed

Pica-Dilly Cheez

Process in food processor adding enough water slowly for desired consistency.

In Food Processor add:

2 cups of pre-soaked sunflower seeds
Juice from 2 fresh squeezed limes
2 cloves of garlic
1 tablespoon/15 mL of dried dill
1 teaspoon/5 mL of mustard powder
1 teaspoon /5 mL of capers
1 teaspoon/5 mL of white pepper
Water, add as needed

Mexicali Cheez

In Food Processor add:

2 cups of pre-soaked macadamia nuts
Juice from 2 fresh squeezed lemon
1 tablespoon/15 mL of nutritional yeast flakes
1 tablespoon /15 mL of garam marsala
1 tablespoon/15 mL of onion powder
1 tablespoon/15 mL of garlic powder
1 tablespoon/15 mL of chili flakes
1 tablespoon/15 mL of cayenne pepper
Water, add as needed for desired consistency

Process in food processor until desired consistency is achieved.

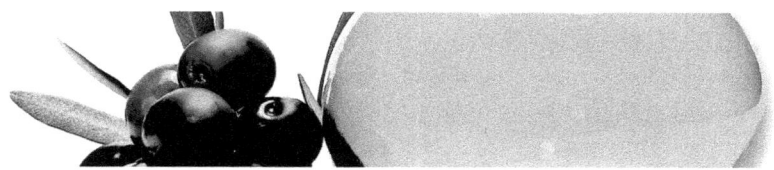

Dressings, Sauces & Condiments

A MUST-ARD Mustard

Blend until puree like consistency, and serve! You can double this mixture as it keeps 4 weeks in fridge, I like small amounts and fresh, the mustard is actually spicy strong when first made, then mellows with each day that passes. Fantastic with sauerkraut on onion bread! So if you like it hot! Make and serve fresh!

In Blender add the following ingredients:

1 cup/250 mL of mustard seed soaked
2 tablespoons/30 mL of nama shoyu
8 Pitted Soft Dates
1/4 cup/60 mL of lemon juice
1 teaspoon/5 mL of miso paste

CATCH UP! Ketchup

Blend until puree like consistency, the sundried tomatoes will act as thickener. Serve chilled, I prefer to make a small amount and serve fresh, try it with our recipe Veggie Nofries! Store the rest in a glass jar and keep in fridge for a few days.
In Blender add the following ingredients:

2 Medium vine-ripened organic tomatoes
1/4 cup/60 mL of apple cider vinegar with mother
2 tablespoons/30 mL of Braggs amino
2 tablespoons/30 mL of Yacan Syrup
2 cloves of garlic
1-1 and 1/2 cups/250-375 mL of sundried tomatoes
2 teaspoons/10 mL of sea salt
2 teaspoons/10 mL of fresh squeezed lemon

Ranch Dressing Avocado

This will make a bottle to store in the fridge for up to 4 days.

Avocado Ranch Dressing is a thicker dressing you may want when serving a salad that contains winter vegetables like cabbage, broccoli, cauliflower etc. You can use this one too as a dip!

In blender add the following ingredients:

1 ripe organic avocado peeled and pit removed
1 organic cucumber peeled and seeded
1/2 cup/125 mL of Extra Virgin, cold pressed olive oil
Juice from one lemon
2 cloves of garlic
Sea salt and pepper to taste

BERRY LEGAL Raspberry Vinaigrette

This will make a bottle to store in the fridge for up to 4 days.

Blend until all ingredients well blended, store in glass decanter in fridge, serve chilled! Enjoy.

In blender add the following ingredients:

1/2 cup/125 mL of Cold Pressed Extra Virgin Olive Oil
1/2 cup/125 mL of red wine vinegar
1/2 cup/125 mL of fresh raspberries
2 tablespoons/30 mL of stevia
2 teaspoons/10 mL of Dijon mustard
1 tablespoon/15 mL of poppy seeds
1/2 teaspoon/2 mL of dried oregano
Add sea salt and black pepper to taste

ORANGE YOU HAPPY? Orange Vinaigrette

In blender add the following ingredients:

1/2 cup/125 mL of fresh squeezed orange juice
1/4 cup/60 mL of Cold Pressed, Extra Virgin Olive Oil
1/4 cup/60 mL of hemp oil
3 tablespoons/45 mL of apple cider vinegar with mother
2 teaspoons/10 mL of raw honey or agave syrup

Sea salt and pepper to taste
Top dressing with a sprinkle of hemp seeds
- This is nicely suited to spinach salads with mandarin oranges.

This delightful citrus dressing will make enough to store in a bottle to store in the fridge for up to 4 days.

Portobello Mushroom Gravy

Process all ingredients until smooth. Steam will come out of the top of this blender, but this is still within the allowable temperature of the raw live vegan program. The sun-dried tomatoes and dates will act as thickeners to your gravy. Everyone has his or her own preference of thickness, so feel free to add a little water if a thinner gravy is desired. You can put the gravy into a pie dish and set it in the dehydrator, below the mock turkey roll, or other choice of dish, to keep it warm until you are ready to eat! Be sure to make plenty, as guests will enjoy it on their mock meat dish AND on their vegetables, greedy gravy grubbers!

In Vita Mix Blender add:

1 cup/250 mL of Vegetable Broth
1 cup/250 mL of Portobello mushrooms
1/2 cup/125 mL of tahini
1/4 cup/60 mL of sundried tomatoes
1/4 cup/60 mL of nama shoyu
1/4 cup/60 mL of onions
1/4 cup/60 mL of dates
1/4 cup/60 mL of purified water 1 clove of garlic

YAYYYO Mayonnaise

This will store well for a week in the refrigerator, plan how you will use it, to use it up! Lovely on cucumber or tomato sandwiches, or as a salad base! Or use when serving your "Fish-Fakes", or 'Chicken Little" recipes.

In Blender or in food processor add the following ingredients:

2 cups/500 mL of cashews
1 cup/250 mL of coconut water
1/2-3/4 cup/125-200 mL of freshly squeezed lemon
2 tablespoons/30 mL of apple cider vinegar
2 soft-pitted dates
2 tablespoons/30 mL of olive oil
1 tablespoon/15 mL of mustard
2 teaspoons/10 mL of sea salt
1 teaspoon/5 mL of onion powder
1 clove of garlic or 1 teaspoon/5 mL of garlic powder

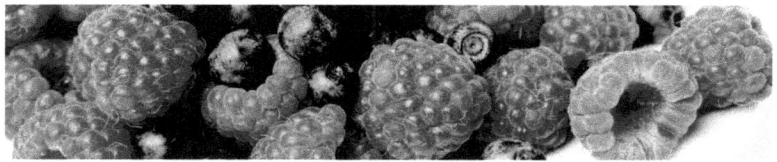

Deserts

Wild Blueberry Crumble Recipe
Serves 6

    3 Cups/750 mL of Wild Organic Blueberries
    6 Tbsp./90 mL of No. 2 Maple Syrup

Step One, Crumble Base
Soak for six hours:

    1/4 cup/60 mL of Buckwheat Groats
    1/4 cup/60 mL of Oat Groats
    1/4 cup/60 mL of Pearl Barley
    1/4 cup/60 mL of Kamut

After grains have plumped up from soaking, spread grains out on teflon lined rack and Dehydrate for 6-8 hours. Set aside. This is a step that could have been done the night before.

Step Two, To make Crumble:
In Food Processor Process add the following ingredients:

    1 cup/250 mL of pre-soaked/dried Almonds
    1 cup/250 mL of Dates
    1 teaspoon/5 mL of Cinnamon
    6 cups of Dehydrated grains

Pulse the ingredients to mix thoroughly.

Assembly:
In individual bowls place:

    1/2 cup/125 mL of blueberries
    1/2 cup/125 mL crumble
    Top with 1 tablespoon of No. 2 Maple Syrup, stir and serve!

Crumble stores nicely in fridge for 4 days. I keep blueberries separate and use Maple Syrup when ready to serve, this way crumble does not get too soggy, but stays crisp!

Chocolate Pudding

Dress your pudding up with toppings, cacao nibs, crushed nuts of your choice, or strawberries! You can also add pure mint extract instead of vanilla and add a mint leave for decoration!

In food processor add the following ingredients and puree until smooth:

   2 ripe avocados
   2 frozen bananas
   2 tablespoons/30 mL of raw cocoa powder
   1 teaspoon/5 mL of seeds from pure vanilla bean
   3 pitted dates

Cinnamon Heart Cookies

This batch can easily be doubled and is very flexible to work with. You can use cookie cutters or you can shape into balls, you can roll them in almond flour or finely ground coconut flakes. These freeze well and do not require to be dehydrated. If you choose to dehydrate to dry them crisper then I recommend no more then 4-5 hours each side. I like them moist, taste the mix and see if you don't agree! If you want ease with cookie cutters a great tip is to work with small amount of cookie dough at a time, roll dough in almond flour or fine raw coconut flakes then place between two layers of parchment paper and use a roller on top of parchment to roll out dough, now use cookie cutters and you will see how easy it is. I don't mind the stickiness of the mix as the end result is a tasty moist cookie! Store in air-tight freezer containers. These cookies store well in the freezer and make for a pretty cookie tray!

In food processor add the following ingredients:

1 cup/250 mL of macadamia nuts
1 cup/250 mL of dates
1 cup/250 mL of raisins
1 tablespoon/15 mL of orange juice
1 teaspoon/5 mL of cinnamon
1 teaspoon/5mL of ginger

Halvah

Halvah Base - In large bowl mix by hand:
1 cup/250 mL of raw tahini
1 cup/250 mL of agave nectar
1 cup/250 mL of raw pistachios
1/2 cup/125 mL of organic cacao powder

Mix together to cookie dough consistency, then spread mixture patting it firmly into square pan. I use an 11X14" pan, but I have also used and 8X8"/12 mm square pan! The smaller pan will give you 1" high 1" square pieces as it is rich, but if you go for larger pan, you will have slimmer larger pieces.

Chocolate Sauce - In Blender add the following ingredients:
1 cup/250 mL of coconut oil
1 cup/250 mL of organic cacao powder
1/2 cup/250mLof maple syrup
1 teaspoon/5 mL or coarse ground sea salt

Assembly of Squares:
Top Halvah base with Chocolate Sauce and freeze to set. Then score squares into 1" squares. Place squares in an air-tight freezer container, separating layers with parchment paper, for storage until serving, serve chilled. Will freeze well for a couple of months. This is a family favourite, family has to be reminded that they must share with company!

Chocolate Almond Bark

On a parchment-lined cookie sheet evenly distribute 1 cup/250 mL of pre-soaked raw whole almonds, that have been towel patted dry. Pour chocolate base over top of almonds, spread around with spatula to get even coat. It does not matter if an almond or two are not covered, they still will be anchored in place by chocolate! Freeze until set, remove almond bark and drop on counter to break bark into pieces. Store in air-tight freezer containers, re-using the parchment paper to layer bark when separating the layers to freeze. This recipe will freeze for a couple of months. Serve chilled!

Chocolate Base- In food processor add:
    1 cup/250mL of coconut oil
    1 cup/250 mL of cacao powder
    1/2cup/125 mL of agave nectar
    1 teaspoon/5 mL of ground coarse sea salt

Caramel Chocolates
Assembly:

Remove candy molds from freezer, Press toffee into molds, fill will remaining chocolate sauce. With a rubber spatula remove excess chocolate from back of mold onto parchment to use in more candy molds or in other recipes. Chocolate Sauce keeps in fridge for about four days. Chocolate Sauce can be used to ice squares, cookies, granola bars, havlah, fruit dip, or top ice cream! Take molds out of freezer an hour or two before serving, set upside down onto parchment paper to release from mold. Nobody will believe you made these by hand! Well worth the effort.

Chocolate Molds:

You will need a deep-set chocolate mold, available at any bulk store. Before beginning this recipe, wash and clean your chocolate mold, dry thoroughly and oil your molds with olive oil and set in freezer while you prepare chocolate sauce.

Chocolate Sauce - In the Food Processor add, do not over process or oil will separate:
   1 cup/250 mL of coconut oil
   1 cup/250 mL of organic cacao powder
   1/2 cup/125 mL of maple syrup
   1 teaspoon/5 mL of sea salt

Remove oil lined candy molds from freezer, oil will be frozen to the mold, pour chocolate into the mold and then tip mold upside down over a piece of parchment paper to let the excess chocolate pour back out, yes out, at this point you are only lining the mold with chocolate. Set mold back in freezer!

Caramel Filling - In Food Processor add the following ingredients:
   1 cup/250 mL of pitted dates
   1 cup/250 mL of pine nuts
   1 teaspoon/5 mL of pure vanilla extract

Process until creamy, toffee like consistency. Shape into tiny balls for deep set round forms or oblong forms for deep set rectangular molds.

Date Squares
Crust Base - In large bowl mix add all the following ingredients:
   2 cups/500 mL of soaked groats (combination of oat groats, buckwheat groats, kamut and barley)
   2 cups/500 mL of oat flakes
   1 cup/250 mL of almond flour
   1/2 cup/125 mL of raw honey

Mix thoroughly and press 2/3 of mixture firmly into bottom of 10" x 10"/15 mL square pan using anything that would substitute as a "tamper" to press mixture into pan, (a cup/spatula has a good flat base), I favour a glass, place glass in water and then tamp oats into pan, repeat this process, a dry cup will lift oat mixture from pan instead of pressing it down.

Filling - In Food Processor, process:
    3 cups/750 mL of dates
    1 cup/250 mL of raisins
    1/2 cup/125 mL of hot water

Process until mixture has a paste like consistency. Spread onto bottom layer of oat crust mixture. Top Date Mixture with remaining oat mixture and tamp down. Put in dehydrator at 118 degrees Fahrenheit for 6 hours. Enjoy!

Apple Pie
Apple Pie Filling - In juicer blend:
    12-16 apples

Place apple pulp in bowl, set aside.

In food processor chop:
    1 cup/250 mL of dried apples
    1 cup/250 mL of walnuts
    1 cup/250 mL of dates
    1/4 cup/60 mL of maple syrup
    2 teaspoons/10 mL of cinnamon
    2 teaspoons/10 mL of nutmeg

Place the above mixture with the apple pulp and add 1 cup of cranberries and 2 teaspoons of chia, stir and add mixture to crust and top with 1/4 cup of remaining crumb mixture. Place in dehydrator for 6 hours, ENJOY!

Pie Crust - In food processor combine:
    1 1/2 cups/375 mL of walnuts
    1 1/2 cups/375 mL of dates
    1/4 cups/60 mL of cane sugar

Tamp down 3/4 crust mix into pie plate, save 1/4 of crumb mixture for topping.

Creamy Dreamy Ice Creamy

Process all ingredients until smooth. This recipe lends itself to using whatever you have in your pantry that goes well with bananas. You can sweeten with honey or maple syrup or agave syrup. You can add whatever type of soaked nuts you want. You could add pure peppermint as a flavouring with cocoa powder instead of cocoa nibs. Make this to suit your taste buds. You may want to add just a bit of water if it is too thick or you may want to add coconut milk or almond milk. These recipes are just that flexible! Now you know what to do the next time you see ripened bananas on sale, buy them to freeze!

In Food Processor add the following ingredients:

- 2 cups/500 mL of frozen bananas
- 2 tablespoons/30 mL of soaked walnuts
- 2 teaspoons/10 mL of cacao nibs
- 2 teaspoons/10 mL of sucanat
- Seeds of vanilla bean or 1 tsp/5 mL of pure vanilla

Frozen Fruit Pops

Pour fruit puree into ice-pop containers or into little ramekins. Insert a coffee stick or spoon and place in freezer to freeze. The psyllium has no taste, but it has the added advantage of thickening the fruit so that the fruit pop does not melt so quickly and drip!

The adult version is to add 1 cup of sake to the fruit and psyllium mixture and pour into ramekins. Partially freeze to serve more as a sorbet! Caution here to separate from what the little ones may perceive to be a treat, no joke, serious consequences!
In High Speed Blender add the following ingredients:

- 1 cup/250 mL of fruit, assorted or 1 type, you choose!
- 1 cup/250 mL of orange juice or water
- 1 rounded teaspoon/5 mL of psyllium powder that will dissolve in blender, blend until pureed.

Ice Kream Sandwiches

"Rich vanilla ice cream sandwiched between two chocolate wafers, nothing says summer more!"

Chocolate Wafers - In Food Processor add the following ingredients:
1 cup/250 mL cup almond flour
1/2 cup/125 mL soaked raw almonds
1/2 cup/125 mL of pitted organic madjool dates
1/4 cup/60 mL of organic cacao powder
1/2 teaspoon/5 mL of pure vanilla extract
1/2 teaspoon/5 mL of sea salt

Process to dough-like consistency, divide dough into half, set dough aside.

Ice Kream - In Food Processor add the following ingredients:
2 cups/500 mL of raw soaked cashews
2 cups/500 mL of soaked raw macadamia nuts
1 cup/250 mL of coconut water
1/2 cup/125 mL of coconut oil
1/2 cup/125 mL of #2 maple syrup
1 teaspoon of sea salt
Seeds from one vanilla bean

Process to cream-like consistency, set aside:

In muffin pan lined with paper cups drop a scoop full of chocolate wafer dough into bottom and press down to form bottom wafer, then place a dollop of ice cream. Take second half of chocolate wafer mix and roll out between two layers of parchment paper, take round cookie cutter to cut out circle shapes to top off ice cream layer. Cover muffin tins with freezer wrap and wait at least 8 hours to set. Serve frozen, Enjoy!

Chocolate Melts
No appliances required
In large bowl add the following ingredients:

- 2 cups/500 mL of "raw" almond butter
- 1/2 cup/125 mL of raw cocoa powder
- 1/2 cup/125 mL of agave syrup
- 1/2 cup/125 mL of coarsely chopped soaked almonds
- 1 tablespoon/30 mL of coconut oil
- 1 teaspoon/10 mL of coarse sea salt
- 1 organic ripened banana mashed
- Seeds from one vanilla bean

Stir until pudding like consistency and drop by spoonfuls into paper muffin cups. I set paper cups in muffin tins, drop the spoonfuls directly into paper muffin cup. Garnish with a nut, sweetened orange peel, mint leaf, edible flower, etc. Wrap whole muffing tin in freezer wrap. Store in Freezer, serve frozen.

Caramel Chews
In Food Processor add the following ingredients:

- 2 cups/500 mL of soaked almonds
- 2 cups/500 mL of dried pineapple
- 1 cup/250 mL of pitted dates
- 1 cup/ 250 mL of raisins
- 1 tablespoon/30 mL of #2 maple syrup
- 1 tablespoon/30 mL of coconut oil
- 1/2 teaspoon/5 mL of sea salt

Form into 1 inch/2 ½ centimeter balls and set aside.

Coating - In Food Processor add the following ingredients:
- 1/4 cup/60 mL of soaked, dried buckwheat groats
- 1/4 cup/60 mL shredded coconut
- 1/4 cup/60 mL almond flour

Process to fine crumb-like consistency. Roll balls in crumb mixture to coat. Store in freezer. Suck on these delicious morsels frozen, best way I know how to beat the heat! Talk about great food on the go!

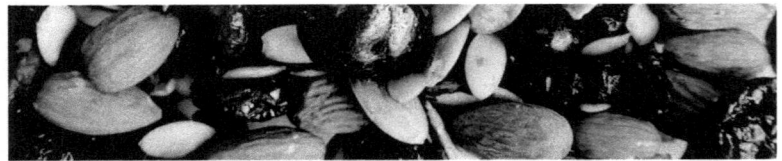

Appetizers & Snacks

Pumpkin Seed Treats Spicy Pumpkin Seeds

Fold seeds so all spices, oil and honey is evenly coated. Spread out onto teflon coated wire dehydrator rack and dehydrate at 118 degrees for 24 hours. It will be hard to not nibble over this time frame!

In bowl add:

> 2 cups/250 mL of drained pumpkin seeds that have soaked for 4 hours in salted water.
> 1/2 cup/125 mL of sunflower seeds
> 2 tablespoons/30 mL of cold pressed olive oil
> 2 tablespoons/30 mL of raw honey
> 1 tablespoon/15 mL of sea salt
> 1 teaspoon/5 mL of chili powder
> 1 teaspoon/5 mL of garlic powder
> 1 teaspoon/5 mL of onion powder

Fold seeds so all spices, oil and hone.

Trail Mix
In Large Bowl toss:

> 1/2 cup/125 mL raisins
> 1/2 cup/125 mL dried apricots
> 1/2 cup/125 mL of dried cranberries
> 1/2 cup/125 mL of dried blueberries
> 1/4 cup/60 mL of dried apples
> 1/4 cup/60 mL pumpkin seeds
> 1/4 cup/60 mL of cacao nibs
> 1/4 cup/60 mL unsalted sunflower seeds
> 1/4 cup/60 mL of pre-soaked dried almonds
> 1/4 cup/60 mL coconut

Sweet Pumpkin Seed Treat

Fold seeds nuts and fruit with sweeteners and spices so all is evenly coated. Spread out onto teflon coated wire dehydrator rack and dehydrate at 118 degrees for 24 hours. The scents of one recipe will not affect the taste of the other recipe if you happen to make both of these recipes and dehydrate at the same time, make both, variety is the spice of Life! Enjoy these spooktacular treats!

In bowl add:

   2 cups/500 mL of drained pumpkin seeds that have soaked for 4 hours in salted water.
   1 cup/250 mL of soaked almonds
   1 cup/250 mL of raisins
   1/4 cup/60 mL of dried cranberries
   1/4 cup/60 mL of large coconut flakes
   1/4 cup/60 mL of maple syrup
   1 teaspoon/5 mL of cinnamon
   1 teaspoon/5 mL of ginger
   1 teaspoon/5 mL of sea salt

Stuffed Mushroom Caps

24 crimini mushrooms (set aside caps after removing stems)

Blend the ingredients and scoop into mushroom, take mushrooms with cheese filling and dip into crushed flax crackers.

In Food Processor add:

   Stems from crimini mushrooms
   2 cups/500 mL of pre-soaked sunflower seeds
   1 tablespoon/15 mL of nutritional yeast flakes
   1 tablespoon/15 mL of nama shoyu
   1 teaspoon/5 mL of minced garlic
   1 teaspoon/5 mL of sea salt

Stuffed Snow peas

Place the ingredients in a food processor, you may require water to get desired consistency add only 1 tablespoon at a time, you do not want it too runny yet not too chunky.

In Food Processor add:
- 2 cups/500 mL of pine nuts
- 2 cloves of garlic
- 1 tablespoon/15 mL of nutritional yeast flakes
- 1 teaspoon /5 mL of garam marsala
- 1 teaspoon/5 mL of cumin
- 1 teaspoon/5 mL of lemon juice
- 24 large organic snow peas (open on seam to form mini boats for stuffing)

Hummus

Blend all of the ingredients in food processor to creamy like consistency, serve.

In Food Processor add:
- 2 cups/500 mL of soaked chick peas, thoroughly rinsed
- 2 cloves of garlic
- juice from fresh lemon
- 2 teaspoons/10 mL of sea salt
- 2 teaspoons/10 mL of chili flakes
- 1 teaspoon/5 mL of garam masala
- 1 teaspoon/5 mL of onion powder
- 1 teaspoon/5 mL of nutritional yeast flakes

Bean-less Hummus

Place the above ingredients in food processor for light chop just enough to blend the ingredients into a creamy consistency.

In Food Processor add:
- 1 Zucchini chopped
- 1/2 cup/125 mL of soaked cashews
- 1/4 cup/60 mL of tahini sauce
- 5 cloves of garlic
- 2 tablespoons/30 mL of hemp oil

Juice from fresh lemon
2 teaspoons/10 mL of sea salt
1/4 teaspoon/60 mL of cayenne pepper
1 jabanero pepper
1/2 teaspoon/2 mL of garam marsala

Salsa

Place the above ingredients in food processor for light chop just enough to mix ingredients.

In Food Processor add:

4 organic sun-ripened tomatoes
1/2 cup /125 mL of Spanish onion
5 jabanero chili peppers
1/2 cup/125 mL of celery
1/4 cup /60 mL of raw corn kernels off the cob
1/4 cup /60 mL of green pepper
1 tablespoon/15 mL of fresh squeezed lemon
1 teaspoon/5 mL of sea salt
1 clove of garlic

Sweet Potato and Kale Chips

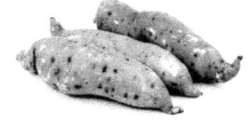

1-2 sweet potato's
   (2 would fill 10 racks of your dehydrator)
1-2 heads of kale
   (2 would fill 10 racks of your dehydrator)

You can use a variety of vegetables though, including beets!

Preparation:

Vegetables like Kale will need the woody back spine removed. Kale is curly and will not lay flat, this is great though as it will take on its own characteristics. The only appliance required to prepare Kale Chips is a sharp knife, cutting board and the dehydrator! Remember chips SHRINK when dehydrated, so a whole leaf divided into quarters may start out at a 3" radius and end up dehydrated a 1" chip!

Sweet Potato and Beet Chips require a mandolin to finely slice them into fine thin slices. You may have a food processor that has a blade, but depending on how wide the feeder spout is, your chips will be very small, so this is why the open concept of a mandolin is the favoured appliance. I do not peel the skin as the skin has its' own nutrients and added fiber! Wash your beets and Sweet Potato and start slicing!

Citrus Oil Coating:

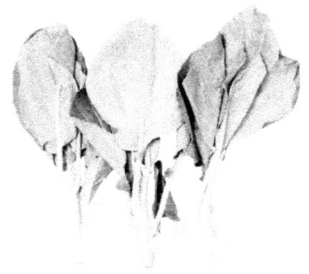

All your vegetables prior to dehydrating require a light coating of Organic olive oil and organic lemon and a dash of sea salt all mixed in a bowl before laying out not overlapping on a teflon coated wire rack. Remember less is more, the vegetables only need a rub, not saturated. The oil and lemon juice can be mixed and placed in food-grade oil spray pump canister available from any kitchen supply centre. Best tool is the Vegetable Spinner, place oiled veggies in spinner to remove excess oil, oil can be re-introduced to oil bottle.

Seasonings:

After kale gets a rub/spray of olive oil and lemon, dust with sea salt, lay out on teflon coated rack and sprinkle nutritional yeast from beet vegetable source, instead of from barley grain source if you are concerned over gluten. If gluten is not an issue then nutritional yeast from barley is fine. Place in dehydrator at 118 degrees Fahrenheit for 5 hours, then turn over onto wire rack, removing the teflon sheet and re-season if necessary and dehydrate for another 5 or until desired crispness is reached.

After sweet potato and beet chips get a rub/spray of olive oil and lemon, then place single layer so that they do not overlap on a teflon coated rack and are then sprinkled with a spice mix, pre-mixed for ease of 1 tablespoon/15 mL each of garlic powder, sea salt, cumin, chili powder. Place in dehydrator at 118 degrees Fahrenheit for 12 hours. Remove rack after 12 hours and turn sweet potato and beet chips over onto open wire rack, and return to dehydrator for another 20 hours or more, the longer they are in the dehydrator, the crisper they will get, I have left them in for 72 hours! Make plenty, these chips will not last long!

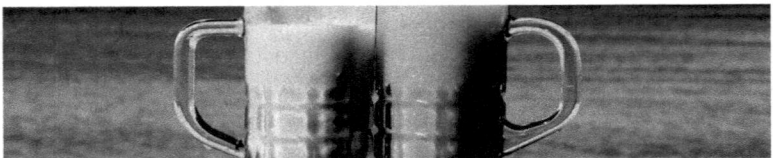

Beverages
Blueberry Smoothie

For added roughage/fiber add 1 tablespoon/15 mL of ground flax or psyllium husk.

In Blender add:

- 1 cup/250 mL of almond milk
- 1 cup/250 mL of frozen wild blueberries
- 2 pitted medjool dates

In blender, blend until frothy, enjoy chilled!

The After Party Juice
Serving for 2-3

TIP: You can also transfer the entire juice into a blender and add the softened Kelp and any other leafy greens (spinach, celery) to it, to add fibre to your juice. This juice keeps in the fridge for 2-3 days.

This juice is most beneficial the morning after a party, as the body naturally will try to alkalize all of the acidic party foods and drinks one has consumed. The calcium present in the leafy green vegetables will restore the body's possibly depleted calcium, and the beets will help cleanse the liver. Thus the name, "The After Party Juice!"

Pour hot water over Kelp to help soften it and make it easier to feed through juicer.

In Juicer add:

- 1 head of broccoli
- 4-5 stalks celery
- 1 cucumber

Handful of spinach
1/4 head of cabbage
1 bunch parsley
4-5 leafs Kale
1 piece Sea Kelp (8"x 3")
1 large beet

The Alkalizer!

L-Glutamine can be purchased at any health food store or body building supplement shop or on-line, I purchase many supplements from *Puritan's Pride* an on-line vitamin/supplement company that offers great deals, buy 2, get 3 free! Willard Water can be purchased at any health food store or on-line!

In Blender add:

1 cup/250 mL of purified water
1 tablespoon/15 mL of L-glutamine powder
1/2 teaspoon of Willard Water
Juice from 1 fresh squeezed lemon

Stir and drink, this is great for increasing alkalinity! Soothes upset stomach.

Almond Milk

Blend until smooth, will store in fridge for 5 days, use in cereal or just as a refreshing drink!

- The remaining pulp from almonds can be used in a cheez recipe!

In Blender add:

1 cup/250 mL of pre-soaked almonds
3 cups/750 mL of water

Blend the above and pour into mesh bag or cheese-cloth bag over bowl squeezing the bag to extract all of the juice. Pour extract back into blender and add the following:

Seeds from 1 vanilla bean(cut bean lengthwise and scrape seeds with sharp knife)
3 pitted medjool dates

Chocolicious Smoothie
In blender add:

1 cup/250 mL of almond milk
1 organic banana
1 tablespoon/15 mL of organic cacao
2 pitted medjool dates

Blend until frothy, enjoy chilled!

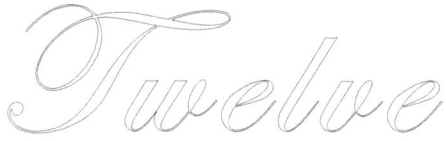

In Closing

Open Yourself to The Possibility

Life presents opportunities when we least resist change. One only has to free their mind and be open to its' possibilities. How many times have we looked for something that we have clearly defined in our head, only to trip upon it unawares and yet know that this is exactly what we were thinking and wanting? Some would shrug it off as coincidence, when actually it is the result of putting positive energy out there. The combination of being clear with what you want and actively looking for it sends vibes out into the universe to deliver. Skeptics would say this is hogwash. Others, who are devout in their beliefs, may say God helps those who help themselves. Regardless of your belief system you cannot argue that there isn't something larger at play here. I count myself as fortunate to have witnessed opportunities over and over again in my life. And I do believe there is a higher power that delivers. I will share a few of the connections and opportunities that have presented themselves to me and you can decide for yourself.

The first opportunity all started with a book. I was enjoying a planned get away to Chester, Nova Scotia for my husband's 50th birthday. We stayed at a five star inn with a dining room and gorgeous accommodations with lovely walkout balconies that extended over the outdoor dining patio. Our evening started on the patio where we met an interesting family. We chatted with them for a while, before returning to our room to sit on our balcony and enjoy a glass of wine and the warm evening before dinner. The conversation below was lively and entertaining, and it seemed as if we had never left. Quietly we enjoyed a father discussing John Guare's play, *Six Degrees of Separation* with his family, explaining that we are all only separated in this universe by six people. He went on to explain that in theory, if one took the opportunity to mingle at a party and engage in conversation with complete strangers the chances of someone knowing someone or finding that common ground would surface at that time. This intrigued me to the point where I bought the book 'Six Degrees of Separation' and read it. My own experience has shown me that it works. The world truly is a small place. It becomes smaller when we are willing to take that first step beyond our comfort zone.

The Six Degrees of Separation experience in my family started with my son, Bryan. Bryan had a close friend in high school. They hung out at each other's houses quite often. When my son became seriously ill, it was my son's friend's mother who came and talked to me about the possibility of contacting Dr. Timmins at BioHealth Diagnostics. Bryan was so ill that his liver was shutting down and as Dr. Timmins was a renowned nutrition specialist, she thought he could help him. Someone who knows someone who could help! My son followed a rigid detox diet eliminating, refined processed foods as well as all dairy and red meat. The family as a whole ate a diet comprised mostly of organic fruits and vegetables and whole unprocessed grains giving his liver time to heal. There is no known pharmaceutical to treat an overburdened liver. The only approach was a strict nutritional holistic one. We sent samples of saliva and excrement in specially prepared vials off to the BioHealth Diagnostic Lab for feedback on his internal health. My son healed rapidly, completed high school, and then went off to University. I, on the other hand, was still suffering the aftershocks of almost losing a son and not having time to deal with it, even though I was grateful for his recovery.

While one of the courses Bryan studied at university was philosophy, I occupied myself relearning everything regarding healthy nutrition, as many of the things I thought were healthy were not. Bryan came home one weekend and observed me busying myself with everything and with nothing, needing to squeeze every last second out of a day. He posed the question, "What would happen if you just stopped and just let yourself be?" I stopped for a moment, totally perplexed at the philosophical words coming from my son's mouth. Tears brimming, I managed, "I think I would explode!" These words hit hard. They drove home the point that I had not allowed myself time to deal with my emotions while my son had been so sick. I had avoided a deep- rooted fear of loss. And there was Bryan wanting to share his interest in philosophy with me by posing a simple philosophical question and I did not see it for what it was. My son was not challenging me, but my frustrated response surprised us both. It also gave me something to think about. A week hadn't passed when surfing through the channels one afternoon I happened upon Oprah's interview with Eckhart Tolle just as he mouthed the words, "Learn to let yourself be!" There they were - those same words, spoken by an intellect on T.V. The same words my freshman son had brought home from his philosophy class in university. Again, driven by the desire to know and understand, I ordered Eckhart Tolle's book, *A New Earth*. It helped me learn more about myself. It also helped me learn to let go, to move on and to engage in life. This book started my fascination with spirituality and search for a clearer picture of our purpose in this life. I enjoyed many books by Wayne Dyer and Rhonda Byrne and their teachings on spirituality. These books tell us that we are all capable of greatness if we only free ourselves to the possibilities. The teachings state that if we are very clear on the things we want, the Universe will deliver. I will share a few events that have occurred in my life and you can decide for yourself.

In my past I had been afflicted with bilateral pterygiums, a small pearl-like growth on the surface of the eye. It developed when I was 21 years old. The pterygiums left my eyes itchy and dry. The camera picked up on this portraying me inevitably as tired. I had a specialist tracking the pterygiums. Here in Canada they use a stitch method to cut out and sew the eyeball leaving the eye messier than they are with the pterygiums in place. But a surgery would have to take place before vision is interrupted. The specialist tracked the pterygiums for over 30 years, waiting for them to travel over my iris so the stitches would be less noticeable. The success rate for the procedure performed here in Canada, a cut and stitch method, was not high, as re-growth can occur. Since becoming a nurse and doing shift work under fluorescent lights my eyes are more red than usual. A fellow nurse asked me one day what a pterygium was and what caused this condition. I had grown accustomed to people asking me what was wrong with my eyes as the pterygiums had become quite noticeable. Having access to a computer, I keyed in the word "pterygium" and up popped an audible screen announcing breaking news PBS posted on the Harvard Eye Clinic in California performing pterygium removal, showing before and after pictures of a non-stitch technique with a 95% success rate in no re-growth and clear eyes. This was a new breakthrough procedure in dealing effectively with pterygiums. I could not believe what I was witnessing. I shared my findings with my husband and contacted the clinic. I asked Dr. Hovanesian, the physician who perfected this technique, and he agreed to take me on as a client. I booked the appointment for nine months down the road, as I needed time to save for the procedure. The surgery took place four years ago and was a complete success as there are no signs of re-growth. I have since had Lasik surgery, which corrected my vision to 20/20, not bad for 53!

Another incident worthy of mention occurred as I neared my 50s. I was peri-menopausal, gaining weight, lacking energy thanks to depleted hormones, and at wits end when trying to get the help I had read about that was available to women my age. I was aware through the media and books that advances were being made to assist women in this area with bio-identical hormones. Unfortunately most of these treatments were available only in the larger cities and not in rural Nova Scotia, or so I thought! One of the books I read suggested searching "compounding pharmacies" with my geographical location on the Internet. I did so and found Moffatt's Drug Store in Dartmouth, Nova Scotia, which is not only a compounding pharmacy, but also gave me the name of Dr. William LaValley who is an American doctor working in Chester, Nova Scotia as well as in his home state, Texas. Chester is less than thirty minutes from my home. I was ecstatic knowing I would not have to travel to Chicago in hopes of seeing Prudence Hall - the hormone specialist. Dr. LaValley was here all along.

After realizing optimum health, I found myself wanting to share the steps my husband, Phil, and I took to achieve our success. Dr. LaValley was very encouraging with my desire to get the message out and www.rawlivevegan.com was created. Through this site I met two more dynamic people, Glenna Jenkins an editor and Elizabeth Hardy a book designer, both interested in the Raw Live Vegan lifestyle and the benefits it offers. Neither ladies knew each other, yet both saw the opportunity and shared my interest and assistance in what has become the book *Living the Raw Live Vegan Lifestyle*. And the rest is history!

The last incident I will share had one more personal issue that needed to be addressed and that was vein surgery. Left untreated, it could lead to a deep vein thrombosis, a silent killer. Knowing health is our wealth and not wanting all of my hard work to be in vain, no pun intended, I decided to have it treated. Having been referred to a vascular surgeon five years previously and still waiting, I took it upon myself to check out vein therapies via the Internet to see if there were any private clinics that could speed up the process. My research led me to www.atlanticveinclinic.ca. This clinic hosted Dr. Matz, who specializes in Endovenous Laser Therapy (EVLT). This procedure first isolates the source of the problematic vein via ultrasound. This was a superior procedure to vein stripping. Had I been called by the specialist for vein stripping, I would have been hospitalized, been anesthetized for the procedure, a known risk, been laid up for a week and in pain. Interestingly enough I had done research on this technique a few years earlier and the closest clinic to my home was in Toronto. At that time, I had to make a choice between the pterygium removal or the vein surgery as they were both costly procedures that required travel. I chose the pterygium removal and put off the vein surgery until 2011. To my delight, it is now available in Halifax, Nova Scotia. Things have a way of presenting themselves to us at the right time. Dr. Matz and his well-organized team performed the painless procedure in March 2011, all while treating me to a movie as this technique did not require anything more than local anesthesia, which is less risky than being put under. Prior to the procedure the leg was mapped with the use of ultrasound to locate and isolate the problematic vein. A tiny

In Closing

catheter containing a laser is then inserted into the vein. The laser energy damages the vein walls shrinking them and closing the faulty vein so that blood cannot flow through it. This eliminates vein bulging at its source as well as the accompanying symptoms such as heaviness, aching, pain, cramps, swelling and numbness. Typically the procedure takes 45 to 60 minutes. I was also told to walk immediately afterward. No down time, as in the week required after vein stripping. And the only pill required was ibuprofen. EVLT has a 98% success rate. I was pre-measured for compression stockings, which I had to wear for 12 hours a day for four weeks post-op, and then only for my 12 hour shifts as a nurse or for doing anything strenuous. Thank goodness beaching is not strenuous!

The few incidents I have shared still amaze me as I think of how and when they unfolded. For me the Universe does deliver, at the right time, and for this I am very grateful! I hope you too will open yourself to the possibilities!

Bibliography

Books listed provided worthy information that has been instrumental in helping me to get where I am today. I believe each person's situation to be unique and urge the reader to consult with a qualified health professional when implementing a raw live vegan lifestyle. The information presented in this book is in no way intended as medical advice or as a substitute for medical counseling, but is meant only as information to guide you in being your own health advocate! I do not advocate the use of any particular diet or exercise program but wish only to share what seemed to be a miraculously speedy recovery to optimal health for not just me but for my husband too!

Clement, Brian R. & Digeronimo Theresa Foy - *Living Foods for Optimum Health*. - New York: Three Rivers Press, a division of Random House, 1st paperback edition 1998.

Hotze, Steven F. M.D. - *Hormones Health and Happiness*.- New York: Wellness Central, Hachette Book Group USA, 1st edition 2005.

Stephenson, Kenna, M.D. - *Awakening Athena*. - Texas: Health, Heart & Mind Institute, 1st edition 2004.

Northrup, Christiane, M.D. - *The Wisdom of Menopause*. - New York: Bantam Dell, revised edition 2006.

Turner, Natasha, N.D. - *The Hormone Diet*. - Random House of Canada, 1st edition 2009.

Vanderhaeghe, Lorna R., M.S. & Pettle, Alvin, M.D. - *Sexy Hormones*. - Markham Ontario: Fitzhenry & Whiteside Limited, 1st edition 2007.

Delaney, Brian M., Walford, Lisa - *The Longevity Diet. Philadelphia*: Da Capo Press, A Member of the Perseus Books Group, 1st edition 2005.

Baroody, Dr. Theodore - *Alkalize or Die*. - North Carolina: Holographic Health Press, 1st edition 1991.

Robert O. Young Ph.D., & Shelley Redford Young - *The pH Miracle*. - New York: Warner Books, 1st edition 2002.

Howell, Dr. Edward - *Enzyme Nutrition*. - Avery a member of Penguin Putnam Inc., 1st edition 1985.

Soria, Cherie, & Davis, Brenda R.D., & Vesanto, Melina, M.S., R.D. - The Raw Food Revolution. - Tennessee: Book Publishing Company, 1st edition 2008.

Soria, Cherie - *Angel Foods*. - Tennessee: Book Publishing Company, revised edition 2003.

Calabro, Rose Lee - *Living in the Raw*. - Tennessee: Book Publishing Company, 1st edition 1998.

Shannon, Nomi & Duruz Sheryl, *Raw Food Celebrations*. - Tennessee: Books Alive, an imprint of Book Publishing Company.

Shannon, Nomi - *The Raw Gourmet*. - Tennessee: Books Alive, 1st edition 1999.

Crocker, Pat - *The Juicing Bible*. - Toronto: Robert Rose Inc., 2nd edition 2008.

Dale Figtree – *The Joy of Nutrition*, book and DVD, www.dalefigtree.com

BioHealth Diagnostics & Dr. William G. Timmins: www.biodia.com. *The Status of Food Enzymes in Digestion and Metabolism*, also by Edward Howell, originally published in 1946, and republished as *Food Enzymes for Health and Longevity* (Lotus Press, 2nd edition, 1994).

Somers, Suzanne - *Breakthrough, Eight Steps to Wellness*.- New York: Crown Publishers, 1st edition, 2008.

Somers, Suzanne - *Ageless, The Naked Truth about Bioidentical Hormones*. - New York: Crown Publishers, 1st edition 2006.

Sources: *Determining & Testing Hormone Levels.* Kenna Stephenson, MD in www.womeninbalance.org

John Guare – a play - *Six Degrees of Separation*. – Vintage Books, Random House, New York, second edition, 1994.

Eckart Tolle – *A New Earth* – "Awakening to Your Life's Purpose." – Plume Group Printing, first edition, September 2006.

Eckart Tolle – *The Power of Now* – Namaste Publishing, Canada, first paperback edition, September 2004.

Rhonda Byrne – *The Secret* – Atria Books, New York, first edition 2006.

Koebnick, Corinna; Garcia, Ada L; Dagnelie, Pieter C; Strassner, Carola; Lindemans, Jan; Katz, Norbert; Leitzmann, Claus; Hoffmann, Ingrid (2005). *"Long-Term Consumption of a Raw Food Diet Is Associated with Favorable Serum LDL Cholesterol and Triglycerides but Also with Elevated Plasma Homocysteine and Low Serum HDL Cholesterol in Humans,2"*. Journal of Nutrition 135 (10): 2372. PMID 16177198

Bibliography

Websites

www.natuopathyworks.com
http://chetday.com/quinoa.html
http://www.bodyecology.com/07/04/12/quinoa_benefits_guide.php
http://lifestyle.iloveindia.com/lounge/benefits-of-quinoa-6494.html
http://www.isga-sprouts.org/history.htm
http://www.sproutpeople.com/grow/harvest.html
http://www.wholisticresearch.com
http://www.soymilkquick.com/benefitofwheatgrassjuice.php
http://www.naturalnews.com/028042_babies_BPA
http://www.findings.net/supremarin.html
http://www.webmd.com/diet/features/superfoods-everyone-needs
http://www.foodmatters.tv/Health_Resources/Green_Superfoods
http://www.best-juicer-reviews.com/benefits-of-juicing.html
http://en.wikipedia.org/wiki/Body_mass_index

Author's Background

Growing up in the sixties, I witnessed many changes in the food industry, and the effects these changes had on our health. It has become my personal obsession to understand and undo this damage by making better nutritional choices. As a nurse, with a background in teaching healthy weight loss management, one would think that I would never have a health issue. But, like many, I slowly succumbed to exposure to additives, preservatives, and processed foods. Even though this was limited, it was enough to leave me in a less than optimal state of health.

Weight wise, my husband and I have always been within the suggested 'normal' range. When we turned 50, health issues related to family genetics became a concern. For my husband, this included a lack of energy, sore joints, increased cholesterol and blood pressure, and a few extra pounds. As far as libido goes, that taboo subject, let's just say he was more tired than usual! When he went for his annual physical, his health problems began to surface.

I, on the other hand, had gone from the bottom of the recommended weight range, for my age and height, to the top, over a matter of 10 years. Added to this was the stress of moving into peri-menopause (now there's a time bomb), and not knowing when I would be transitioning from peri to flat out menopause! But, as my blood pressure was good, my cholesterol was low, and my thyroid checked out fine, my doctor gave me a clean bill of health. According to him, there was no need to worry until my waistline exceeded 35 inches and I had topped the weight range for my age and height! In

Author's Background

his estimation, I was the picture of perfect health for a woman my age.

I was unhappy with our doctor's 'wait and see' approach to health, for Phil and I. This doctor's care was guided by parameters and ranges set by modern medicine. When a patient does not fit within these ranges, they are prescribed a drug to "manage" the condition. I knew, then, that we had the wrong doctor.

Our idea of optimal health is to be active in our elder years and as opposed to being relegated to the sidelines. Also, considering my husband's current health issues and my own, I felt that time was of the essence. I pushed on, attending conferences on cutting edge health topics, reading, and watching endless documentaries on health-related environmental issues. I also sought a doctor gifted in health issues related to aging to serve us as clients.

Serendipity occurs when one accidentally stumbles upon something wonderful, when searching for something else. This serendipitous moment, for us, occurred during the pursuit of optimum health. After searching for solutions to my and my husband's health problems, I found Dr. William LaValley. This doctor was versed in cutting edge medicine and believed in both natural and pharmacological remedies, depending on the specific health issues of the client.

At present, my husband and I practice 80% raw live vegan. But, my advice to anyone starting out is to transition into the program, by introducing one raw meal at a time.

Enjoying the healthful gains and benefits, over a year and a half of a raw live vegan lifestyle, encouraged me to create rawlivevegan.com! I am so passionate about my project that it no longer feels like work! It is my personal wish to teach

Author's Background

you the importance of "real-whole- organic food" and the life-long benefits they provide. Hopefully, you will pass on this vital information, so that your loved ones will also benefit from the nurturing and healing qualities of raw food.

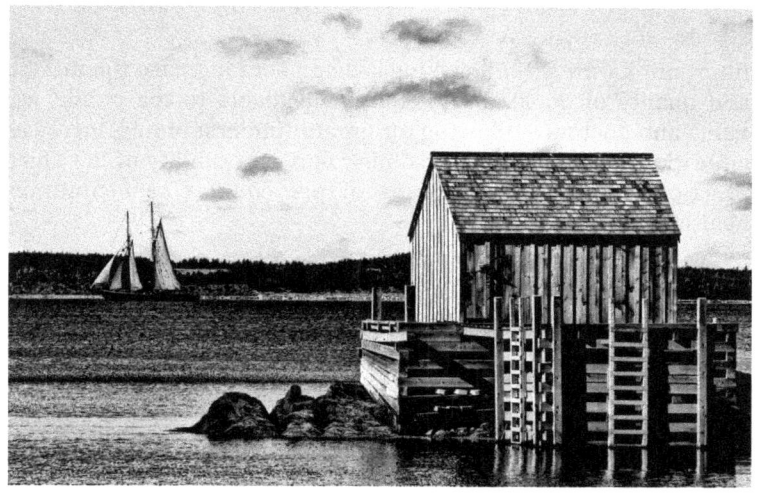

Dr. J. William LaValley
227 Central Street
Chester, Nova Scotia
Canada. B0J 1J0
totalhealthbreakthroughs.com

Dr. Jeoff Drobot
200, 110 Point Mckay Cres.
North West Calgary, Alberta
Canada. T3B 5B4
calgarynaturopathic.com

Dr. Dena Churchill
2684 Oxford Street,
Halifax, Nova Scotia
Canada. B3L 2V1
drdenachurchill.com

INTERNATIONAL HEALTH PUBLISHING

Inspiring readers of the world to experience the light. International Health Publishing books express truth and wisdom, encourage spiritual enlightenment, facilitate growth and healing – while also providing a phenomenal reading experience.

International Health Publishing's vision is to increase the number and quality of books and resources available to the public, students and doctors – allowing for greater understanding, increased education, as well as more visibility and accessibility of the Chiropractic profession as a means of preventative and continued health care.

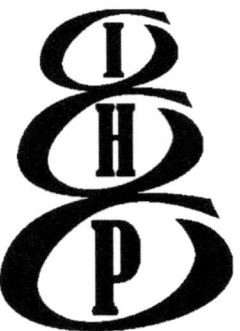

INTERNATIONAL HEALTH PUBLISHING
Adjusting and Growing
International Headquarters • Carrollton, Texas

www.InternationalHealthPublishing.com

www.ingramcontent.com/pod-product-compliance
Lightning Source LLC
Chambersburg PA
CBHW071314150426
43191CB00007B/621